Love: A Melanated Skincare Guide

Copyright © 2025 by Lakischa Morgan

All rights reserved.

Permission to reproduce or transmit in any form or by any means, electronic or mechanical, including photocopying, photographic and recording audio or video, or by any information storage and retrieval system, must be obtained in writing from the author.

Love: A Melanated Skincare Guide is a registered trademark of Lakischa Morgan.

First printing February 2025

Paperback ISBN: 979-8-218-61779-0

Published by Royal Palms Publishing, LLC
Eva Myrick, MSCP, Publisher

Printed in the U.S.A.

Love: A Melanated Skincare Guide

LAKISCHA MORGAN

Disclaimer

The information provided in *Love: A Melanated Skincare Guide* is intended for general knowledge and educational purposes only. It is not a substitute for professional medical advice, diagnosis, or treatment. The skincare tips, routines, and product recommendations in this book are based on personal experiences, research, and knowledge in dermatology; however, individual skin conditions vary, and results may differ from person to person.

Before beginning any new skincare regimen, please consult a qualified dermatologist or healthcare provider, especially if you have underlying health conditions, allergies, or specific skin concerns. The author and publisher are not liable for any adverse effects, allergic reactions, or other health issues resulting from the use of information or products mentioned in this book.

This book does not endorse any specific products or brands and is intended to share guidance to help readers make informed decisions about their skincare. Always perform a patch test before using new products to ensure compatibility with your skin.

By reading this book, you acknowledge that you are responsible for your own skincare choices and that this book serves as a resource to guide you on your skincare journey.

TABLE OF CONTENTS

Introduction iii

Chapter 1
Understanding the Anatomy of Your Skin 1

Chapter 2
The Science of Melanin 7

Chapter 3
Understanding Your Skin Type 13

Chapter 4
What Is a Dermatologist? 23

Chapter 5
Exploring Common Skin Conditions 33

Chapter 6
Common Myths 53

Chapter 7
Building a Solid Foundation: The Essentials of a Good Skincare Regimen 55

Chapter 8
Revealing Radiance – A Guide to Retinol for Melanated Skin 61

Chapter 9
The Magic of Moisturizing for Melanin-Rich Skin 71

Chapter 10
 SPF, SPF, SPF! 77
Chapter 11
 Feed Your Skin: The Power of Nutrition and Health for a Balanced Life 83
Chapter 12
 The Sun, Vitamin D, and Melanin Skin 89
Chapter 13
 Embracing Youthfulness: A Melanated Guide to Anti-Aging 93
Conclusion 97
Acknowledgements 99

Introduction

This may come as a surprise, but our skin is actually an organ. In fact, it is the largest organ in the human body, and for melanated people, it carries not only beauty but also heritage, culture, and resilience. Yet, when it comes to skincare, many of us have found ourselves overlooked, frustrated, or confused by a sea of products and advice that just don't seem to work. *Love: A Melanated Skincare Guide* began with my own similar journey in 2012, through the highs and lows of caring for my own skin and helping others throughout my dermatology career.

In a world filled with countless skincare routines, beauty products, and the latest cosmetic trends, my professional journey has always centered around one goal: helping people feel confident in their skin. As someone who has faced skin challenges myself, I know just how transformative a healthy complexion can be. So, it may come as no surprise that I didn't just stumble into dermatology; I pursued it with passion, education, and a commitment to guiding others through the sometimes overwhelming world of skin health. My background is a blend of both medical and cosmetic expertise, giving me a unique perspective that goes beyond what many skincare enthusiasts encounter.

Through my education, I learned the science behind skin health and how our largest organ responds to various internal and external factors. Working on the medical side gave me insight into how conditions like acne, hyperpigmentation, rosacea, and more affect people not only physically but emotionally. There's an undeniable confidence that comes from healthy, clear skin, and I wanted to help others experience that. Over the years, I've worked with dermatologists, estheticians, and countless clients, building my expertise in treatments ranging from acne solutions to anti-aging regimens.

As I immersed myself deeper into the field, I recognized that medical knowledge alone wasn't enough. To create truly transformative skincare experiences, I needed to understand the art of beauty and wellness. This led me to the Aveda Institute, an institution renowned for its emphasis on holistic skincare and the power of natural ingredients. My training there as an esthetician broadened my skill set, helping me appreciate the balance of science and artistry that goes into creating beautiful skin. At Aveda, I learned how to apply principles of relaxation, nourishment, and rejuvenation, which are just as important as clinical treatments. These experiences allow me to create customized, comprehensive skincare routines that targeted each of my client's unique needs.

My passion has always been to educate and empower. Over my career, I've had the privilege of helping thousands of people, from those struggling with lifelong skin issues to those simply wanting a refreshed, radiant glow. Each person I've worked with has taught me something new, and with each success, I am reminded of why I chose this path. I understand the frustration that can come from trying product after product or the emotional impact that acne, cysts, or scarring can have on someone's life. My approach to skincare is deeply empathetic because I've been there myself. I know what it's like to deal with breakouts, search for answers, and finally find solutions that work.

As folks with melanated skin, we often face unique challenges—hyperpigmentation, dryness, oiliness, and sensitivity—while navigating an industry and world that hasn't always recognized our needs. Through this guide, my hope is to provide you with the tools, knowledge, and most importantly, the confidence to love and care for your skin with intention.

This quick guide is designed to be your trusted companion as you discover what works for you. Through this book, I aim to pass on the knowledge I've gained from years of experience, study, and practice. We'll begin by discussing the science of skin, providing you with foundational knowledge on why we care for our skin the way we do. Next, we'll dive into some common skin conditions you may be dealing with and how to treat them, debunk some skincare myths, and uncover a basic skincare regimen that benefits most skin types. Finally, I'll leave you with specific guidance on how to use retinols, moisturizers, and SPF effectively, and explain how our skin is impacted by both our internal and external environment.

Whether you're just starting out on your skincare journey or you're looking to refine your regimen, my hope is that you'll feel equipped and inspired to take the steps needed to achieve the skin you desire. The tools and techniques I share come from both science and heart, honed over years of dedication to this craft. Skincare isn't just a job for me; it's my calling, my purpose, and my way of helping others find confidence in the skin they're in.

This book isn't just about routines and products, though those are important. It's about celebrating the rich diversity of melanated skin and empowering you to take charge of your skincare with love, patience, and pride. Whether you're struggling with finding the right routine, tired of battling skin issues, or simply looking to enhance your natural glow, this guide is for you. Let's embark on this journey of self-love, self-care, and healing together because you deserve it!

With love and light,
Morgan

Chapter 1:

Understanding the Anatomy of Your Skin

Before embarking on any kind of skincare journey, it's important to gain a brief understanding of the structure of the skin so you can make sense of its unique needs and challenges and work with it—instead of against it—to achieve a healthy, radiant glow.

The Skin's Three Main Layers
Think of the skin as an ecosystem with different layers and elements working together to protect, hydrate, and regenerate themselves. Our skin is composed of three main layers: the epidermis, dermis, and hypodermis (or subcutaneous layer). Each layer plays a critical role in maintaining skin health and appearance.

The Epidermis: Your Protective Barrier
The outermost layer of the skin, the epidermis, is the first line of defense against the world. This layer is what we see when we look in the mirror, and it's also where the skin's regeneration and protective functions take place. Pretty much every step of a skincare

regimen addresses the epidermis in one way or another to promote health and vitality.

Cleansing and moisturizing target the epidermis by cleaning and hydrating the skin to maintain its barrier function and health. Treatments, such as serums with active ingredients, may penetrate slightly deeper but still work within the epidermis and exfoliation works to remove dead skin cells, improve texture and tone, and promote cell turnover, which allows your skin to maintain a healthy glow.

The epidermis itself has several sub-layers, with each one contributing to the skin's barrier function:

- Stratum Corneum: This is the topmost layer, often referred to as the "skin barrier." It consists of dead skin cells packed tightly together with natural oils. This layer works to keep moisture in while blocking out harmful substances like dirt and pollution.

- Stratum Lucidum (Clear Layer): This layer is found only in thick, hairless skin like the palms of the hands and soles of the feet, providing an additional layer of protection and reducing friction in areas of the body that experience high wear and tear.

- Stratum Granulosum (Granular Layer): In this next layer, cells undergo a process called keratinization, which prepares them to protect the deeper layers. Here, lipids (fat) are also released to form the skin's water barrier, preventing dehydration.

- Stratum Spinosum (Prickly Layer): Just above the basal layer, this layer provides strength and flexibility to the skin. Like the stratum granulosum layer, cells here start to produce keratin, a protein critical for skin integrity. Langerhans cells, which help with immune responses, are also present here.
- Basal Layer: This is the deepest part of the epidermis, where new skin cells are produced. As these cells mature, they move up through the layers of the epidermis, eventually reaching the surface and shedding off. This process is essential for skin renewal and repair.

Together, these layers contribute to the protective and regenerative functions of the epidermis. The epidermis often has a higher concentration of melanin, the pigment responsible for skin color, than deeper layers of skin. Melanin not only determines skin tone but also provides some natural protection against UV damage. However, this doesn't mean we're immune to sun damage; SPF and limited sun exposure are still crucial.

The Dermis: Where the Magic Happens

Beneath the epidermis lies the dermis, a thicker, more complex layer that's home to many of the skin's most vital structures. This is where we find collagen and elastin fibers—proteins that give our skin its firmness and elasticity. When we talk about "anti-aging" products or treatments that promote firmness, they're mainly targeting the dermis. In the dermis, we also have:

- Blood Vessels: These vessels supply oxygen and nutrients to the skin and carry away the body's waste products. Good circulation is essential for a healthy, radiant complexion.

- Sebaceous (Oil) Glands: These glands produce sebum; an oily substance that helps moisturize and protect the skin. Overproduction of sebum can lead to acne, while underproduction can result in dryness and flakiness.
- Sweat Glands: Sweat glands help regulate body temperature and aid in detoxifying the skin. They also play a role in maintaining the skin's pH balance.

The Hypodermis: Cushioning and Insulation

The hypodermis, or subcutaneous layer, is the deepest layer of the skin, primarily made up of fat and connective tissue. This layer acts as a cushion, protecting our internal organs and bones from injury and insulating the body to maintain a stable internal temperature. Most topical skincare products and routines are designed to address the epidermis and, to some extent, the dermis, but not the hypodermis. This skin layer is just too deep for these products to penetrate.

Massage, facial tools like gua-sha, and techniques like microneedling can stimulate circulation in the hypodermis to increase blood flow and promote collagen and elastin production. Tattoos are designed to reach the dermis, but not the hypodermis. If tattoo needles penetrate too deeply into the hypodermis, it can lead to uneven ink deposits, pain, or even scarring.

The Skin Barrier and Why It Matters

The skin barrier is a physical structure, and its condition reflects the overall health and quality of your skin. The skin barrier, also called the stratum corneum, is the outermost layer of your skin made up of skin cells and lipids (fats). Its main job is to lock in moisture to keep your skin hydrated and supple and keep out any irritants, bacteria, and pollutants that could harm your skin or cause infections elsewhere in the body. In melanated skin, maintaining a healthy barrier is especially important because our skin can be more sensitive to external triggers, leading to issues like hyperpigmentation when it is compromised.

Technically, you can see and touch the skin barrier because it's the outermost layer of your skin. However, its health and function aren't always visible to the untrained eye. When the skin barrier is weakened—often due to harsh products, environmental factors, or even stress—the skin can become chronically dry, flaky, irritated, inflamed, and more susceptible to breakouts, while an intact barrier generally looks smooth and feels soft.

To support a strong barrier, avoid over-exfoliating, which can strip away natural oils; moisturize regularly to replenish and maintain hydration; and use gentle, pH-balanced cleansers that don't disrupt the skin's natural acidity (I provide recommendations for cleansers in chapter 2).

Skin Types and How Anatomy Plays a Role

The anatomy of your skin, particularly in the epidermis and dermis layers, influences your unique skin type. We'll dive deeper into each skin type in chapter 3, but for now, here's a quick overview of how different elements contribute to the most common skin types:

- Oily Skin: Often caused by overactive sebaceous glands in the dermis. Proper cleansing and balancing products can help manage excess oil without stripping necessary moisture.
- Dry Skin: Results from a weakened barrier in the epidermis, which allows moisture to escape more easily. Focus on hydrating products and avoid ingredients that may further dehydrate the skin.
- Combination Skin: Some areas of the face, like the T-zone (forehead, nose, and chin), may have more active sebaceous glands, resulting in oilier skin, while other areas are drier, often requiring a tailored routine.
- Sensitive Skin: The skin's barrier can be more fragile, leading to increased reactivity with certain products. Choosing mild, hypoallergenic products is crucial.

Understanding the anatomy of your skin can allow you to make more informed choices in your skincare regimen. By taking care of each layer and supporting your skin's natural functions, you'll be better equipped to manage issues like acne, dryness, or hyperpigmentation in a way that respects your skin's unique makeup.

Chapter 2

The Science of Melanin

The beauty of melanin-rich skin lies in more than its outward glow; it also carries the remarkable legacy of human evolution, adaptation, and resilience. Melanin is a pigment that occurs naturally in human skin, hair, and eyes. In scientific terms, melanin is produced by cells called melanocytes, which reside in the skin's outer layer (the epidermis). There are two primary types of melanin: eumelanin, which gives skin a darker brown or black hue, and pheomelanin, which produces lighter shades that look more red or yellow.

Melanin production is triggered when melanocytes synthesize melanin to absorb and dissipate ultraviolet (UV) radiation from the sun. This is why people with higher levels of melanin in their skin are naturally more protected against UV damage. As humans evolved, the presence of melanin-rich skin became an evolutionary advantage, particularly for those who lived near the equator, where sunlight was more intense and constant year-round. Don't get too excited, though. It is still best practice to apply sunscreen each day to fortify your skin's protection against harmful UV rays.

The Evolution of Skin Color

Around 200,000 years ago, the earliest humans evolved in East Africa. The intense, direct sunlight in these regions necessitated a natural protection mechanism against harmful UV rays, which prompted the skin to produce more melanin. This adaptation was essential for survival, as it shielded the skin from UV-induced DNA damage and minimized the risk of sunburn. The melanin-rich skin of our ancestors allowed them to thrive in the sun-drenched lands they called home.

As humans migrated out of Africa and into areas with less sunlight, such as Europe and Northern Asia, the need for melanin-rich skin decreased. With less sunlight available, the body struggled to synthesize adequate vitamin D, which is crucial for bone health and immune function. Consequently, lighter skin became advantageous in these environments, as it absorbed more UV light, allowing people to produce the necessary amount of vitamin D. This gradual change over millennia shows how our skin tone is an evolutionary masterpiece, adapting to our environments in response to the body's needs.

The Purpose of Melanin Beyond Protection

While melanin's most immediate function is to protect the skin from UV radiation, it has other protective roles as well. Melanin functions as an antioxidant, helping to protect cells from oxidative stress, a type of cellular damage linked to aging and various health conditions. Additionally, melanin can neutralize free radicals, which are unstable molecules generated by UV exposure, pollution, and other environmental stressors that can also cause damage to necessary cells, protein, and DNA. Left to roam freely in the body, free radicals and oxidative damage can lead to a variety of health problems, including accelerated aging; chronic diseases, like diabetes, arthritis, Alzheimer's, and Parkinson's; an increased cancer risk; and a weakened immune system.

In a holistic sense, melanin's protective properties reveal that it is more than just a defense mechanism. For generations, people with melanin-rich skin have lived in environments that demanded resilience and adaptability, so it should come as no surprise that melanin-rich skin carries an inherent strength, a story that reflects humanity's capacity to adapt, protect, and overcome.

Our skin has long been cherished and celebrated by various cultures. In many ancient societies, people recognized the value of darker skin as a blessing bestowed by nature. African and Indigenous cultures around the world regarded melanin-rich skin as a sign of beauty, health, and vitality—and many still do today. In these cultures, skin tone was often linked with the strength to endure the elements, a connection with the earth, and the divine itself. The reverence for melanin-rich skin has deep roots and has transcended generations, carrying symbolic meaning that still resonates today.

In modern times, melanin-rich skin continues to be a source of pride and identity. With a broader understanding of the biology behind melanin, people with melanin-rich skin have come to celebrate not only their skin's beauty but also its unique origin and role in humanity's survival.

Caring for Melanin-Rich Skin

Melanin-rich skin may be inherently protected from some UV radiation, but it still requires care, respect, and nourishment, especially in modern environments where pollution, diet, and stress impact skin health. Acknowledging our skin's history means honoring it with the right balance of protection and care and recognizing that a consistent skincare routine is not just about beauty but about embracing the legacy written in our skin.

Although everyone's skin, regardless of the amount of melanin, needs to be cared for properly, there are certain things that folks with melanin-rich skin should consider ensuring their skin remains in its healthiest state. These differences aren't necessarily about what is needed but rather the degree of focus we should put on certain steps.

1. Gentle Cleansers: Melanin-rich skin is more prone to irritation and post-inflammatory hyperpigmentation (PIH), meaning harsh cleansers can exacerbate dark spots or uneven skin tone. To combat this, use sulfate-free, pH-balanced cleansers that remove impurities without stripping the skin.
2. Consistent Moisturization: Melanin-rich skin may have a more robust barrier function, which can sometimes lead to dryness and an ashy appearance if not properly hydrated. Look for moisturizers with humectants, like glycerin or

hyaluronic acid, and emollients, like shea butter or ceramides, which work to lock in moisture.

3. Sun Protection: A common misconception is that melanin-rich skin doesn't need sunscreen. However, melanin doesn't fully shield us against UV damage, which can worsen hyperpigmentation and lead to premature aging. Use a broad-spectrum sunscreen with at least SPF 30 daily, preferably one that doesn't leave a white cast (I provide some SPF recommendations in chapter 10).

4. Treatment for Hyperpigmentation: Melanin-rich skin is more likely to develop dark spots after inflammation, acne, or injury. Ingredients like niacinamide, azelaic acid, or kojic acid can help brighten skin and even out its tone. Retinoids are also effective but should be used cautiously to avoid irritation.

5. Avoid Over-Exfoliation: Over-exfoliating can trigger sensitivity or PIH. Use chemical exfoliants like lactic acid or mandelic acid, which are gentler on melanin-rich skin, no more than one to two times per week.

6. Tailored Products: The natural oil production in melanin-rich skin can vary, often leaning toward combination or oily. Choose non-comedogenic products to avoid clogging pores while providing necessary hydration.

Melanin is more than a pigment; it's a reminder of the resilience and adaptation that defines us. For every dark spot, freckle, or shade we carry, there is a history, a science, and a story. The origin of melanin-rich skin is a testament to survival and adaptability, a legacy that honors those who came before us and the environments that made us who we are. Through understanding, we deepen our appreciation, creating a foundation not only for beauty but for the pride that comes from knowing our past and embracing our skin's unique, powerful heritage.

Chapter 3

Understanding Your Skin Type

Knowing your skin type is foundational in creating an effective skincare routine. Each type has unique characteristics and challenges, and using the wrong products can either be ineffective or make existing issues worse. In this chapter, I'll explain the main skin types, share advice on how you can identify yours, and offer some tips for managing it effectively.

The Five Basic Skin Types
Most skincare professionals categorize skin into five main types: normal, oily, dry, combination, and sensitive. While everyone's skin is unique, and there are some variations, these categories offer a helpful starting point for understanding how your skin functions and what products or treatments can be most effective in giving you the results you're looking for.

Before we dive in, it's important to note that skin type is not entirely static and can change over time due to various factors such as age, environment, lifestyle, and skincare routine. While genetics play a significant role in determining your baseline skin type, external and internal influences can alter its behavior. For instance, hot and humid weather often makes skin oilier, while cold and dry conditions can lead to dryness and flakiness. Environmental toxins can clog pores and irritate the skin, potentially increasing sensitivity. And over time, sun damage can cause dryness, roughness, or even skin thinning.

Additionally, as we age, our skin tends to produce less oil, making it more prone to dryness. Younger skin may be more likely to lean oily, while mature skin often becomes dry or sensitive. I'm sure many of us have experienced the increase in oil production as we moved through puberty in our teen years. And finally, our diet, lifestyle, and medical conditions all play a role in how our skin behaves during various stages of life. Drinking plenty of water helps maintain skin's elasticity and hydration, while consuming excessive sugar or processed foods can lead to inflammation and breakouts. Certain treatments, like acne medications or steroids, can make skin drier or more sensitive, and issues like eczema or rosacea can alter skin behavior, making it more prone to irritation.

Again, while your baseline skin type may not change entirely, its condition and behavior can shift depending on various external and internal factors. Adapting your skincare routine to meet these changing needs is key to maintaining healthy, balanced skin.

Normal Skin
Characteristics:
- Well-balanced, with neither excess oil nor dryness
- Even tone and smooth texture

- Small, less visible pores
- Few breakouts or blemishes

Skincare Tips:

- Stick to gentle, balanced products to maintain the skin's natural health.
- Keep hydration a priority but avoid overly oily products that may upset the skin's natural balance.
- Incorporate a sunscreen, a gentle cleanser, and a light moisturizer into your routine.

Oily Skin

Characteristics:

- Shiny appearance, especially in the T-zone (forehead, nose, and chin)
- Larger, more visible pores
- Prone to blackheads, whiteheads, and acne

Skincare Tips:

- Look for oil-free and non-comedogenic products to reduce clogged pores and breakouts.
- A salicylic acid cleanser can help exfoliate and clear excess oil from the skin.
- Use a lightweight, oil-free moisturizer to keep skin hydrated without adding extra shine.

Dry Skin

Characteristics:

- Flaky, rough patches, especially in cold weather
- Tightness or sensitivity, particularly after washing
- Fine lines may be more visible, even at a young age

Skincare Tips:

- Hydrating cleansers and rich moisturizers are essential to keep dry skin nourished.
- Avoid products with alcohol or harsh ingredients that can strip away natural oils.
- Try using a hydrating mask and adding a facial oil to your routine to lock in moisture.

Combination Skin

Characteristics:

- Oily in the T-zone but dry or normal in other areas
- Enlarged pores in oily areas with smaller, less visible pores elsewhere
- Can experience occasional breakouts, often around the nose and chin

Skincare Tips:

- Use products formulated for combination skin or target different areas with different products.
- Light, gel-based moisturizers work well in the T-zone, while richer creams can be used on drier areas.

- Exfoliate gently to prevent clogged pores in oily areas without irritating dry patches.

Sensitive Skin

Characteristics:
- Easily irritated, often red or itchy after trying new products
- Prone to redness, burning, or stinging sensations
- May experience conditions like rosacea or eczema

Skincare Tips:
- Avoid products with fragrance, alcohol, and other potential irritants.
- Look for gentle, hypoallergenic, and fragrance-free formulas.
- Patch-test any new products on a small area of skin before applying them to your face.

How to Determine Your Skin Type

If you're unsure of your skin type, try this simple test:

1. Wash your face with a gentle cleanser and pat dry.
2. Wait for an hour without applying any products, allowing your skin to return to its natural state.
3. Observe how your skin feels and looks. If it feels balanced and comfortable, you likely have normal skin. If it's shiny all over, you probably have oily skin. If it feels tight or has flaky areas, you likely have dry skin. If it's shiny in some areas and

dry in others, you probably have combination skin. If it feels irritated, red, or itchy, you may have sensitive skin.

Embracing My Combination Skin

When I first started my skincare journey, I had no idea what "combination skin" even meant. Like most teenagers, I just knew my T-zone could get as shiny as a glazed doughnut by midday, while the rest of my face—especially my cheeks—often felt dry and tight. What baffled me even more was how stubborn this pattern was. No matter what I tried or how much I experimented with my skincare routine, my skin remained relatively the same over the years: oily in some places, dry in others, and consistently a puzzle to figure out.

Combination skin is exactly what it sounds like—a mix of different skin types on different parts of your face. For me, the oily areas primarily include my forehead, nose, and chin, while my cheeks tend to be dry to normal. It's a skin type that requires balance, and achieving that balance has been both a challenge and a journey for me.

Back then, my approach to skincare was chaotic: overly harsh cleansers, random moisturizers that clogged my pores, and scrubs that left my skin irritated. I treated my oily areas as though they were the enemy and completely neglected the needs of the dry parts of my face. It took years for me to understand that combination skin isn't something to "fix." It's a type that simply requires extra care and a tailored approach to keep it healthy.

The breakthrough came when I started focusing on balance rather than control. I learned that my skin's needs weren't at odds with each other; they just needed specific, targeted care. Instead of treating my whole face the same way, I began thinking of my skincare routine as two mini routines in one.

For my oily T-zone:

- I use gentle, foaming cleansers to remove excess oil without stripping my skin.
- Lightweight, non-comedogenic moisturizers are key; hydration is just as important for oily skin as it is for dry skin.
- Blotting papers and mattifying primers help control shine during the day without clogging my pores.

For my dry areas:

- Richer, creamier moisturizers ensure my cheeks stay hydrated and smooth.
- I incorporated hydrating serums with ingredients like hyaluronic acid to plump and soothe my skin.
- Once or twice a week, I use a nourishing overnight mask for added moisture.

Over the years, I've noticed that my skin's behavior has remained fairly consistent. My T-zone is still prone to oiliness, especially during the warmer months, while my cheeks tend to get drier in the winter. What has changed is my ability to manage it effectively. Combination skin might be tricky, but it's not impossible to care for. The key is listening to your skin and adjusting your routine based on its needs. I've also learned to embrace the quirks of my skin type. The oiliness in my T-zone means I'm less prone to premature wrinkles in that area, while the dryness on my cheeks reminds me to prioritize hydration.

Through the years, my combination skin has taught me patience and acceptance. It's a reminder that no one has perfect skin, and that's okay. Skincare isn't about achieving flawlessness; it's about nurturing your skin and appreciating its unique needs. Combination skin may have its challenges, but it's also resilient, adaptable, and beautiful in its own way. And for that, I've learned to be grateful.

My Advice for Combination Skin

If you have combination skin like me, here's what I'd recommend:

1. Double Cleanse: Use a gentle oil-based cleanser to remove makeup and sunscreen, followed by a water-based cleanser to clean your skin without stripping it.
2. Multi-Masking: Apply clay masks to your oily areas and hydrating masks to your dry areas at the same time. This approach saves time and addresses your skin's specific needs.
3. Don't Skip Moisturizer: Even if your T-zone feels oily, you still need to hydrate. Look for lightweight gels for oily areas and richer creams for dry patches.

4. Sunscreen Is Non-Negotiable: Protecting your skin from UV damage is crucial, no matter your skin type. opt for a sunscreen that won't clog your pores or leave a greasy residue.
5. Be Patient: It can take time to find the right balance, but consistency is key. Stick to a routine and adjust it as needed.

Tailoring Your Routine to Your Skin Type

Knowing your skin type helps you select the right products, but remember that skin can also change due to factors like age, hormones, seasons, and even stress. Pay attention to how your skin reacts and adjust your routine as needed. By understanding your skin's needs, you're setting the foundation for a healthier, more radiant complexion. The next step? Learning how to manage common concerns specific to your skin type, which we'll cover in the following chapters.

Chapter 4

What Is a Dermatologist?

Before moving onto common skin conditions and treatments you can use to combat them, let's talk a little about the professionals who are here to help you achieve your skin goals: dermatologists. When you're struggling with your skin, it can be confusing to know where to turn, especially with so much (often contradicting) information online. Friends, family, and social media influencers might offer advice on what's worked for them, but skincare isn't one-size-fits-all. This is why it's important to consult dermatologists. They're trained experts who specialize in skin, hair, and nails, and they're equipped to address everything about your unique skincare needs, from simple skin concerns to complex medical conditions.

Understanding Dermatology

Dermatology is the branch of medicine that deals specifically with skin, hair, and nails. Given that skin is our largest organ, its health is crucial not just for appearance but for our overall well-being. Many people treat skin conditions as isolated problems, something to be solved with a cream or cleanser. But more often than not, what we see on the outside is a signal that something deeper is happening within the body. Skin conditions can act as warning signs, alerting us to potential underlying health issues that require attention. For example, what you see on the outside as acne and persistent breakouts could be a sign of hormonal imbalances, gut health issues, or increased stress. And your bothersome eczema could be sign of immune dysregulation, allergies, or even nutrient deficiencies.

In my own journey, I've come to realize that my skin is my body's way of communicating with me. Whether it's a breakout around my period or dry patches during stressful times, my skin reflects the state of my overall health. By listening to these signals and addressing the underlying causes, I've not only improved my skin but also my overall well-being. Your skin is your ally, not your enemy. Pay attention to what it's trying to tell you; it just might lead you to a healthier, more balanced life. If you're having a hard time figuring out what's going on with your skin, your dermatologist will be able to guide you down the right path.

A dermatologist's primary role is to help people achieve and maintain healthy skin, using both their clinical expertise and the latest science. Whether it's acne, eczema, psoriasis, or skin cancer screenings, dermatologists are highly trained medical professionals who specialize in diagnosing and treating conditions related to the skin, hair, nails, and mucous membranes. This emphasis on the medical side of things is what differentiates a dermatologist from an esthetician, or someone you may go to for beauty treatments like facials. While estheticians are also licensed professionals, dermatologists are medical doctors who have successfully completed four years of medical school and three to four years of a specialized residency. Because of this, dermatologists are uniquely qualified to offer common treatments like facials, dermaplaning, and microneedling, but they can also perform medical procedures like biopsies, skin cancer removal, and advanced cosmetic treatments like Botox, fillers, and laser work.

Seeing a dermatologist can make a profound difference, especially for those who struggle with chronic issues like cystic acne, eczema, or hair loss. These well-informed professionals can also treat more serious conditions like skin infections, certain types of skin cancer, nail conditions, and recurring issues like seborrheic dermatitis, keratosis pilaris, or hidradenitis suppurativa. It may come as no surprise that acne is one of the most common reasons people seek out a dermatologist, especially since it can often leave behind lasting scars and hyperpigmentation. A skin professional can work with you to create a personalized skincare routine, identifying products or treatments that will be effective for your skin type. While drugstore products can help with surface-level issues, persistent problems like this often need more targeted treatment that a dermatologist can provide. For example, dermatologists can prescribe medication or recommend procedures like chemical peels, microdermabrasion, or laser therapy to help reduce cystic or hormonal acne and even out skin tone.

Beyond acne, dermatologists can also help with issues like hair thinning, dry patches, dark spots, and even signs of aging. And above all, they can help you understand the why behind your skin issues, identifying any underlying conditions or lifestyle factors that might be affecting the health of your skin.

Limits of a Dermatologist's Scope
While dermatologists can address many conditions, there are situations where their expertise is limited. If a skin condition is a symptom of a broader issue—such as internal organ dysfunction, systemic inflammation, an autoimmune disease, psychiatric conditions, or nutrition-related issues—a dermatologist may refer the patient to another specialist. For example, skin symptoms like jaundice or spider angiomas may require evaluation by a hepatologist to address liver disease, and skin conditions tied to malnutrition or deficiencies, such as scurvy or pellagra, may require treatment by a nutritionist or internist. Additionally, Advanced Surgical Interventions:

While dermatologists can perform certain skin surgeries on their own, complex cases involving deeper tissues or cosmetic reconstructions may require a plastic surgeon or other specialized surgeon.

In certain instances, it may be worth it for you to seek a different medical professional. For example, if your skin condition doesn't improve with standard dermatological treatments, or if your skin symptoms are accompanied by other signs like fever, joint pain, fatigue, or significant weight changes, it may indicate an underlying systemic issue that requires further investigation by an internist or relevant specialist. Additionally, if skin conditions are causing significant emotional distress, anxiety, or depression, seeking help from a mental health professional can be beneficial.

In conclusion, dermatologists are essential for addressing skin-specific issues, but they often act as the first line of defense in identifying underlying health conditions. When skin symptoms point to something beyond their scope, a collaborative approach with other professionals helps ensure that patients receive the best possible care. If you're unsure which professional to consult, starting with a dermatologist is a good choice; they can guide you to the right specialist if needed.

Dermatologists for People of Color

For Black, Indigenous, and people of color (BIPOC), finding a dermatologist who understands the unique needs of melanated skin is key. As we've discussed, Black and brown skin has its own needs and conditions like hyperpigmentation, keloid scarring, and certain types of acne that can appear differently on darker skin tones. Unfortunately, some dermatologists may not have specialized training or experience with melanated skin, which is why it's important to look for a dermatologist who understands your specific needs and is experienced enough with melanated skin to provide effective treatments that consider your skin's unique structure.

In my own experience, finding the right dermatologist was a journey. As a teenager, I went through countless breakouts and flare-ups, often around my menstrual cycle. I tried everything I could find on the shelves, but nothing seemed to work long-term. When I finally saw a dermatologist, I was introduced to treatments and insights I'd never considered before. For the first time, I felt like I had someone in my corner who understood the battle I was fighting with my skin.

Just as with any health professional, it's important to feel comfortable with your dermatologist. Building a trusting relationship is essential because skin care is deeply personal. Don't be afraid to ask questions, voice your concerns, or share your skincare goals. A good dermatologist will listen and make you feel at ease, even if you're struggling with something that feels as vulnerable as acne or scarring. They're there to support and empower you to love the skin you're in.

Questions to Ask Prospective Dermatologists

Although it can feel time-consuming and labor-intensive, it's important that you properly vet your medical professionals, including your dermatologists, to ensure they'll be able to provide you with the care you're looking for. Here are a few questions you can ask your dermatologist to get a sense of their overall experience, expertise with certain skin conditions, and the progress they've seen in their clients.

- How much experience do you have treating skin of color?
- What percentage of your patients have melanated skin?
- Have you completed additional training or education on treating skin of color?

- How do you approach treating hyperpigmentation or dark spots in melanated skin?
- What treatments do you recommend for keloids, and have you successfully treated them in patients with darker skin tones?
- How do you manage conditions like melasma, eczema, or acne in skin of color?
- Are there any treatments you avoid or adjust when working with darker skin tones, such as lasers or chemical peels?
- Do you use Fitzpatrick skin typing when evaluating a patient's skin?
- Can you share examples of successful treatments with patients who have skin like mine?

The answers and reactions you receive by asking these questions can help you make a decision about whether or not you feel comfortable moving forward with certain professionals. As a general note, if the dermatologist you are talking to doesn't give direct answers or avoids questions regarding expertise, generalizes all skin types without acknowledging the unique needs of melanated skin, and/or recommends treatments known to have higher risks for darker skin (e.g., certain lasers) without clear precautions, it may be in your best interest to thank them for their time and look elsewhere. Being informed and direct during this stage of the vetting process can help you ensure your professional is knowledgeable and capable of addressing your specific skincare needs.

Where to Find Dermatologists

Here, I've provided a few resources and directories that can help you find dermatologists who specialize in melanated skin.

- Skin of Color Society (SOCS): www.skinofcolorsociety.org
    - This organization focuses on research and education related to skin of color. Their directory allows you to search for dermatologists with expertise in treating melanated skin.
- American Academy of Dermatology (AAD): www.aad.org
    - Use the "Find a Dermatologist" tool and filter by specialties like "ethnic skin" or "skin of color."
- Black Dermatologists Directory: www.blackdermdirectory.com
    - This directory lists Black dermatologists across the US who are experienced in treating melanated skin.
- Melanin Skin Health: www.melaninskinhealth.com
    - A platform dedicated to connecting people with dermatologists who specialize in the treatment of darker skin tones.

Social Media & Community-Based Platforms

- Instagram and Tik Tok: Search hashtags like #BlackDermatologist, #SkinOfColorExpert, or #MelanatedSkincare to find professionals showcasing their expertise.

- Facebook Groups and Forums: Join groups like Black Skin Care Advice or Melanin Skin Professionals to get recommendations from others.
- RealSelf (www.realself.com): This site offers reviews and recommendations for skincare professionals, including dermatologists and estheticians, with user feedback on their expertise with melanated skin.

The Power of Professional Support

If you've been struggling to manage your skin concerns on your own, seeing a dermatologist can be the start of a whole new chapter in your skincare journey. Their training, expertise, and access to advanced treatments can bring about significant changes that may feel out of reach on your own. I encourage you to consider dermatology, not just as an option for "serious" cases but as an important, proactive step in feeling your best and achieving your skincare goals.

Chapter 5

Exploring Common Skin Conditions

On the journey to achieving healthy, glowing skin, many of us with melanated skin may face similar challenges, namely hyperpigmentation, eczema, and acne. Each of these issues brings its own set of frustrations and complexities, but the good news is they can be managed with the right knowledge and care.

I know firsthand how difficult it can be to deal with persistent breakouts or patches of dry, irritated skin. In my teenage years, I tried many patches, serums, and cleansers that promised overnight results, and boy was I fooled. However, over time, through research and personal experience, I learned how to manage my skin more effectively. Now, I'm sharing that knowledge with you.

In this chapter, we'll break down what causes the most common skin conditions we may face, and how to identify them, and, most importantly, the steps you can take to manage them. Whether you're dealing with post-acne dark spots, chronic dry patches, or the occasional breakout, I've got you covered. It's time to take control of your skin, starting from a place of understanding and empowerment.

Hyperpigmentation

Hyperpigmentation is one of the most common skin concerns for those with melanated skin, often resulting from acne scars, sun exposure, or even hormonal changes. While melanin-rich skin gives us a natural radiance and protection from some sun damage, it can also be more prone to developing dark spots and uneven tone when irritated.

Hyperpigmentation refers to patches of skin that are darker than your natural skin tone. This happens when melanin—the pigment that gives skin its color—is overproduced in certain areas. Dark spots, post-acne marks, melasma, and age spots are all types of hyperpigmentation that can affect people of all skin tones, but they are particularly visible on darker skin.

For many folks with melanin-rich skin, hyperpigmentation is often triggered by inflammation, which means that any skin condition causing irritation can lead to darker marks. This includes acne, eczema, bug bites, or even over-exfoliation.

Common Causes of Hyperpigmentation

Understanding what causes hyperpigmentation can help you treat it more effectively. Here are the main contributors:

- Post-Inflammatory Hyperpigmentation (PIH): This is one of the most common causes that occurs after any type of skin trauma or inflammation, like a pimple or scratch. PIH can leave behind brown, purple, or red spots, depending on the depth of the inflammation.

- Sun Exposure: UV rays trigger melanin production as a defense mechanism, but without sunscreen, sun exposure can darken existing spots and lead to new areas of hyperpigmentation. This is one reason why it is recommended that everyone wear sunscreen, even those with darker skin tones.
- Hormonal Changes (Melasma): Hormonal shifts, particularly during pregnancy or due to birth control, can lead to melasma, which is a type of hyperpigmentation that often appears on the cheeks, forehead, and upper lip.
- Skin Care Products and Treatments: Strong chemical peels, incorrect exfoliants, or harsh treatments that aren't designed for melanin-rich skin can lead to irritation and hyperpigmentation.

Steps to Treat Hyperpigmentation

Hyperpigmentation can be stubborn, but with consistency and the right ingredients, it's possible to significantly reduce dark spots. Here's a routine designed to fade pigmentation over time. As always, be sure to perform a patch test before using new products to ensure compatibility with your skin.

1. Gentle Cleansing: Start with a gentle cleanser that won't strip the skin or disrupt its barrier. Over-cleansing or using harsh products can make hyperpigmentation worse. Look for cleansers with soothing ingredients like chamomile, aloe vera, or green tea.

2. Vitamin C: This is a powerful antioxidant that brightens skin and fades dark spots by reducing melanin formation. Use a vitamin C serum in the morning to help even skin tone.
3. Niacinamide: Also known as vitamin B3, niacinamide helps even skin tone, improves skin elasticity, and strengthens the skin barrier. It works well with other brightening ingredients and can be used in both morning and evening routines.
4. Alpha Arbutin: Derived from bearberry plants, alpha arbutin is a gentle, effective ingredient for lightening dark spots and evening out skin tone. You can find this ingredient in a number of serums (like The Ordinary Alpha Arbutin 2% + HA), creams (like Naturium Alpha Arbutin Cream 5%) and toners (like Some by Mi Galactomyces Pure Vitamin C Glow Toner).
5. Licorice Root Extract: This natural brightener inhibits melanin production and reduces inflammation, making it especially useful for post-inflammatory hyperpigmentation. You can find this ingredient in cleansers (like CeraVe Hydrating Cream-to-Foam Cleanser), toners (like Klairs Supple Preparation Unscented Toner), serums (like SkinCeuticals Discoloration Defense Serum), essences (like Missha Time Revolution the First Treatment Essence), creams and lotions (like La Roche-Posay Rosaliac AR Intense), and spot treatments (like Mario Badescu Whitening Mask).

6. Retinoids: Retinoids or retinol (a milder form) boost cell turnover and can help fade dark spots over time. Because retinoids can sometimes cause irritation, start with a low concentration, apply every few days, and gradually increase as your skin adapts.
7. Daily Sunscreen: Sunscreen is a non-negotiable in treating and preventing hyperpigmentation. Look for a broad-spectrum SPF 30 or higher to protect against both UV-A and UV-B rays. Mineral sunscreens with a tint are especially helpful for melanin-rich skin, as they won't leave a white cast and can help blend minor pigmentation. I share recommendations for my favorite SPFs in chapter 10.
8. Exfoliation (one to two times per week): Regular exfoliation can help fade dark spots by promoting skin renewal. Look for gentle exfoliants like mandelic acid, which is found in alpha hydroxy acid (AHA) products like serums, toners, peels, and cleansers targeting acne, uneven skin tone, and fine lines. Avoid physical scrubs (products with beads, facial sponges, etc.), which can cause micro-tears in the skin and worsen hyperpigmentation over time.

Professional Treatments for Stubborn Spots

Sometimes, home treatments aren't enough to fully remove dark spots. In these cases, you'll likely need to seek out other treatments to see results. Here are some professional options that can complement your skincare routine. As always, be sure to seek out a dermatologist who is experienced working with darker skin tones.

- Chemical Peels: Mild peels with glycolic, lactic, or mandelic acid can help fade dark spots when done by a professional who understands melanin-rich skin. Overly strong peels can exacerbate hyperpigmentation, so take your time in choosing a reputable dermatologist.
- Microneedling: As the name suggests, microneedling uses tiny needles to create micro-injuries in the skin, stimulating collagen production and promoting skin renewal. This can help heal hyperpigmentation, especially deep-set scars.
- Laser Treatments: Some laser treatments, like Q-switched lasers, can be safe for darker skin and can target pigmentation directly; however, not all lasers are safe, as some can trigger additional pigmentation. Be sure to talk over your options with a qualified professional.

Preventing Future Dark Spots

The best way to deal with hyperpigmentation is to prevent it from occurring in the first place. One of the best things you can do to prevent hyperpigmentation is to avoid picking at your skin. It can be tempting to pick at pimples, but this can make post-inflammatory hyperpigmentation much worse. Let pimples heal naturally and consider using spot treatments (more on this soon) to help them heal faster. It's also recommended that you use sunscreen religiously, as it is your best defense against pigmentation. Apply it daily, even on cloudy days, and reapply it if you're outdoors for extended periods. And finally, build a consistent routine. Consistency is key for both treating and preventing hyperpigmentation. Stick with a routine, and remember that brightening the skin takes time—sometimes months of consistent care.

If you're looking to prevent post-inflammatory hyperpigmentation (PIH) specifically, there are a couple additional things you should consider. One, prioritize regular gentle exfoliation with ingredients like lactic acid or mandelic acid. These gentler AHAs can help fade dark spots without irritating the skin. Keep in mind, though, that over-exfoliation can make PIH worse, so aim to exfoliate only one to two times a week. Brightening serums made with ingredients like vitamin C, licorice root extract, and azelaic acid are also effective in reducing PIH and evening skin tone. These products are generally safe for darker skin tones and won't lead to rebound pigmentation when used correctly.

The Emotional Impact of Hyperpigmentation

Hyperpigmentation isn't just a cosmetic concern; it can have a significant impact on self-esteem. For many women, it's frustrating to deal with persistent dark spots, and the slow progress to lighten them can be discouraging. While my personal experience with hyperpigmentation has been minimal, I've had the privilege of helping thousands of individuals navigate the emotional and psychological toll it often carries. The many years of working in Dermatology, I've seen firsthand how hyperpigmentation can deeply affect someone's self-esteem and become a source of insecurity. I've counseled countless people who felt diminished by the judgment of others, constantly hiding behind makeup or avoiding social interactions altogether.

What I've learned is that healing hyperpigmentation isn't just about the right treatments or regimens; it's about helping people rediscover their worth beyond their skin. I've worked to provide not just solutions but also compassion and understanding, reminding my patients that they deserve to feel confident at every stage of their journey.

Treating hyperpigmentation is a journey, and small changes can make a big difference over time. Be patient with your skin and focus on the other aspects of your skincare that make you feel good. Hyperpigmentation doesn't define you, and there are effective ways to care for your complexion so you can feel confident every day. Remember, every spot and mark is part of your unique beauty, and with the right approach, you can achieve an even, radiant glow that celebrates the beauty of your melanin.

Eczema

Eczema, also known as atopic dermatitis, is a chronic skin condition that causes inflammation, redness, dryness, and itching. It often appears as patches on the skin, which can become cracked and sometimes ooze or become infected. Eczema can occur at any age but is more common in children and people with a family history of allergies, asthma, or other immune-related conditions.

While there's no known cure for eczema, it can be managed with treatments that reduce symptoms and prevent flare-ups:

- Moisturizing: Keeping the skin hydrated is crucial. Use thick creams or ointments (like petroleum jelly) multiple times a day, especially after bathing.
- Avoid Triggers: Eczema can be triggered by various factors, including certain fabrics, soaps, detergents, food allergies, stress, and environmental allergens. Identify and avoid these triggers.
- Topical Steroids: Mild corticosteroid creams can reduce inflammation and itching during flare-ups. For severe cases, stronger steroids or other topical medications may be prescribed by a doctor.
- Non-Steroid Medications: Newer treatments, such as calcineurin inhibitors (e.g., tacrolimus or pimecrolimus), can be used to control symptoms without the side effects of steroids.
- Antihistamines: These can help reduce itching, especially if it disrupts sleep.
- Bathing Practices: Use lukewarm water and gentle, fragrance-free cleansers. After bathing, pat the skin dry and immediately apply a moisturizer to lock in moisture.
- Phototherapy: In some cases, controlled exposure to ultraviolet (UV) light can help manage eczema.

- Oral Medications: For severe cases, oral medications such as systemic corticosteroids or biologics may be recommended by a dermatologist to control inflammation.

If eczema persists despite at-home/over-the-counter treatments, it's best to see a dermatologist for a personalized care plan.

Acne

Acne can feel like an uninvited guest that never leaves. It can pop up at the worst times, seemingly with a mind of its own. But if we dig a little deeper, we find that there are different types of acne, each with distinct causes and behaviors. Acne, in its many forms, is one of the most common skin conditions, transcending skin color. It occurs when hair follicles become clogged with oil, dead skin cells, and bacteria. Acne can show up in various ways, including blackheads, whiteheads, pimples, and cysts. There are different severities of acne, and it can affect people of all ages. However, it tends to peak during puberty and the teenage years when oil production increases.

I've battled with acne as a teenager, and as someone with melanin-rich skin, I know how challenging it is to manage breakouts without risking hyperpigmentation. Throughout my journey, I've tried just about every trick in the book, but I've learned that a gentle but consistent skincare routine is essential, and treating hormonal acne required me to look deeper and make some lifestyle adjustments too. By staying mindful of what's happening internally as well as on the surface of my skin, I've found a routine that lets me feel confident in my skin—even on those challenging breakout days.

In this section, we'll explore the basic causes of acne, factors that contribute to it, how it affects melanated skin, the difference between general acne and hormonal acne, and the best strategies to help manage it. My goal is to empower you with knowledge so you can recognize what type of acne you're dealing with and begin to take control of your skincare journey. Acne, particularly in melanin-rich skin, is often a journey that requires both care and patience. Remember: you are not alone, and with the right approach, you can work toward clearer, healthier skin and find relief.

Basic Causes of Acne

As I previously mentioned, acne is generally caused by clogged hair follicles, but there are a few ways this can take place. First is with excess sebum production. This occurs when your skin naturally produces too much of the oil it needs to stay moisturized. Next is the bacteria Propionibacterium, which thrives in oily skin and causes inflammation and irritation. Dead skin cells can also build up on the surface of the skin and mix with your skin's natural oil, creating blockages. And finally, general inflammation can make acne symptoms worse. When your body detects blocked pores and bacteria, it sends white blood cells to fight the invaders, leading to increased redness and swelling.

In melanated skin, there are additional factors that can contribute to acne:

- Hormonal Fluctuations: Hormones, particularly androgens, can drive oil production, leading to clogged pores. Black women may notice more acne around their menstrual cycle, pregnancy, or during hormonal shifts, such as starting or stopping birth control.
- Genetic Predisposition: If family members struggled with acne or hyperpigmentation, it may make you more prone to these issues.
- Environmental Factors: Pollution and humidity can irritate the skin, aggravating acne for some people.
- Product Sensitivities: Many mainstream skincare products contain ingredients that can be overly drying or irritating for melanin-rich skin. Avoid products with high levels of alcohol, sulfates, or fragrances, as these can lead to inflammation and darkening of the skin.

Why Acne Can Be Different for Black Skin

For those with melanin-rich skin, acne often presents unique challenges, including a higher risk of post-inflammatory hyperpigmentation (PIH) and specific scarring patterns. Although our skin's higher melanin content makes it look rich and beautiful, it also causes it to respond differently to inflammation and trauma.

Common Acne Types in Black Skin

- Papules and Pustules: Small, red, inflamed bumps (papules) or pus-filled pimples (pustules) are common in Black skin. Due to increased melanin, these lesions are more likely to leave dark marks once they heal.

- Cystic Acne: Deep, painful cystic acne can be particularly troublesome, as it is more likely to cause scarring and hyperpigmentation, especially around hormonally sensitive areas like the jawline and chin.

- Keloidal Scarring: While not everyone develops keloids, Black skin can be prone to keloidal scars—raised scars that form when acne lesions heal and produce excess collagen. This type of scarring can make treating acne especially complex and frustrating.

Hormonal Acne

Hormonal acne is a type of acne that's specifically triggered by fluctuations in hormones. For many people, hormonal acne becomes particularly noticeable around the teenage years, but it can also show up later, especially for women due to their unique hormonal cycles and changes, like menstrual cycle, pregnancy, polycystic ovary syndrome (PCOS), and menopause.

The primary hormone involved in acne is androgen, which can increase sebum production. When androgen levels are high, your body produces more oil, and this excess oil can lead to clogged pores and pimples. Androgens are also responsible for the increased oiliness around menstruation and during stressful periods, which can lead to breakouts.

Common signs that your acne may be hormonal include:
- Timing: Hormonal acne often flares up around your menstrual cycle. Many people notice breakouts just before their period, when hormones like estrogen and progesterone drop.
- Location: Hormonal acne is more likely to appear along the jawline, chin, and cheeks. This area is particularly sensitive to androgens, which are hormones that stimulate sebum production.
- Type of Blemish: Hormonal acne often manifests as deep, painful cysts that don't come to a head. These cysts tend to be resistant to traditional over-the-counter treatments and can linger for weeks at a time.
- Adult-Onset: Unlike typical acne, hormonal acne can start or persist well into adulthood. Some women notice that their acne worsens in their twenties, thirties, or even forties, often due to changes in birth control, pregnancy, or menopause.

Effective Strategies for Managing Acne in Melanated Skin
- Gentle Cleansing: Start your routine with a gentle, sulfate-free cleanser that doesn't strip your skin of natural oils. Look for ingredients like salicylic acid or benzoyl peroxide if you

have oily or acne-prone skin, but start with lower concentrations (2% to 5%) to minimize irritation.

- Incorporate Exfoliation Carefully: Exfoliating regularly can help remove dead skin cells that may clog pores, but it's essential to avoid abrasive scrubs that can cause micro-tears, leading to hyperpigmentation. Instead, try a chemical exfoliant containing glycolic acid or lactic acid, which are generally gentler on melanin-rich skin, and limit use to once or twice a week. Salicylic acid is also excellent for acne because it's oil-soluble, meaning it can penetrate clogged pores and clear them out.

- Topical Retinoids: Retinoids help speed up cell turnover and keep pores clear. Start slow, as these can be drying.

- Target Acne with Spot Treatments: For spot treatments, products with tea tree oil, sulfur, or benzoyl peroxide can be effective at killing acne-causing bacteria, but these should be used sparingly to prevent irritation. A newer, more targeted option is to use hydrocolloid patches (pimple patches), which work by absorbing excess oil from cysts or pustules.

- Hydrate and Protect: Hydration is key for all skin types, but it's particularly important for melanated skin, which can lose moisture faster. Use a lightweight, non-comedogenic (pore-clogging) moisturizer daily and follow up with a sunscreen of at least SPF 30.

- Address Hyperpigmentation with Patience: Post-acne dark spots can be managed with ingredients like vitamin C, niacinamide, and alpha arbutin, which help to brighten the skin gradually and prevent new dark spots. Remember, consistency is key, and these treatments may take a few weeks to show visible results.

Effective Strategies for Treating Hormonal Acne

Treating general acne and hormonal acne involves some overlap, but hormonal acne often requires a more targeted approach. Since hormonal acne is rooted in internal causes, the approach includes both skincare and potential hormonal regulation. Here are some options:

- Birth Control Pills: For women, certain birth control pills can regulate hormones and reduce acne.
- Anti-Androgen Medications: Spironolactone is a prescription medication that blocks androgen receptors in the skin, reducing oil production.
- Diet and Lifestyle Changes: Reducing dairy and high-sugar foods, which can spike insulin and androgens, may help. Lowering stress levels can also reduce cortisol, another hormone linked to acne.
- Topical Treatments: Many of the same topicals used for general acne (salicylic acid, benzoyl peroxide, retinoids) can help, but hormonal acne often benefits from a focus on anti-inflammatory and soothing ingredients like niacinamide and zinc.

- Seek Professional Help: For deep cystic acne, see a dermatologist who can provide treatments like chemical peels, cortisone shots, or oral medications.

At-Home Treatments and Natural Remedies

Natural remedies can offer gentle solutions to manage acne, but they should be used with caution. Here are some that tend to work well with melanin-rich skin:

- Aloe Vera: This natural anti-inflammatory can calm irritation and redness. Use pure aloe vera gel as a spot treatment or mix it with a gentle moisturizer to soothe the skin after a breakout.
- Tea Tree Oil: Known for its antibacterial properties, tea tree oil is helpful for spot-treating active pimples. Always dilute it with a carrier oil, such as jojoba oil, to avoid irritation, and use it only on individual pimples rather than across the face.
- Turmeric: With anti-inflammatory and brightening properties, turmeric can help reduce acne and lighten dark spots. Create a mask with turmeric powder and a gentle base like yogurt, but be mindful that turmeric can stain the skin if used in excess.

Over-the-Counter Treatments

If you're looking for effective, non-prescription options, several ingredients and products work well for acne-prone melanin-rich skin.

- Benzoyl Peroxide (2.5% to 5%): Benzoyl peroxide is a powerful antibacterial agent. For darker skin tones, a lower concentration is usually recommended to avoid irritation. Use it as a spot treatment initially and monitor how your skin reacts before applying it over a larger area.
- Salicylic Acid: This beta-hydroxy acid (BHA) penetrates the pores to exfoliate from within, preventing clogged pores and reducing acne. It's less likely to cause irritation or PIH than other acids, making it a great choice for melanin-rich skin.
- Niacinamide: Known for its soothing and brightening properties, niacinamide is excellent for addressing both acne and hyperpigmentation. It helps reduce inflammation, minimizes pore appearance, and fades dark spots, making it an ideal ingredient for darker skin.

Seek Professional Guidance

Consulting a dermatologist who specializes in Black skin can be invaluable, especially if over-the-counter treatments don't seem to work. A dermatologist can help with prescription options, such as retinoids or azelaic acid, which are often highly effective for acne and hyperpigmentation.

For persistent or severe acne, dermatologists can recommend medical treatments that work specifically for melanin-rich skin.

- Topical Retinoids: Retinoids, such as tretinoin or adapalene, are commonly prescribed for acne because they work to increase cell turnover, reduce clogged pores, and prevent breakouts. Retinoids can also help fade hyperpigmentation over time.

- Oral Medications: If topical treatments aren't enough, oral medications like antibiotics, hormonal treatments, or even spironolactone (for hormone-related acne) can help. These medications target acne from within and are particularly helpful for deep cystic acne. It's essential to work with a dermatologist to find the right dosage that minimizes side effects.
- Chemical Peels: When done by a professional, peels like salicylic acid or glycolic acid can be effective for managing acne and hyperpigmentation. However, since melanin-rich skin is more sensitive to PIH, opting for milder peels with a trained professional is crucial.

Lifestyle Tips for Clear Skin

Beyond treatments, our lifestyle choices also play a crucial role in managing acne. Above all, be sure to eat a well-balanced diet, manage your stress well, and stay hydrated inside and out. Studies show that certain foods, like high-glycemic foods and dairy, can trigger acne in some people. While everyone's skin reacts differently, maintaining a balanced diet with fresh fruits, vegetables, and whole grains is beneficial for overall skin health.

Additionally, stress can lead to hormone fluctuations, which can, in turn, trigger breakouts. Incorporating practices like meditation, exercise, or journaling into your routine can be powerful tools to keep stress-related acne at bay. And I'm sure you know just how important it is to drink plenty of water, but you can also help keep acne at bay by using hydrating skincare products that prevent the skin from overproducing oil and clogging your pores.

Every person's skin is unique, so creating a regimen tailored to your specific needs is essential. Begin with gentle, non-irritating products and introduce stronger treatments gradually. For example, start by cleansing with a mild, sulfate-free face wash, then apply a treatment like niacinamide or salicylic acid, and finish with a lightweight, non-comedogenic moisturizer. Listen to your skin and adjust as needed. If something causes irritation, back off or switch to a gentler alternative. Patience is key. Most treatments take time to show results, and consistency is what will bring the most noticeable improvements.

It's worth remembering that both general and hormonal acne take time to treat. For many people, hormonal acne in particular can be persistent and may never completely disappear, but it can be managed. Be patient with yourself, and remember that skincare is a journey. Some products might work wonders for a few months, then seem to lose their effect; this is common with hormonal acne, as hormonal fluctuations can continue to impact the skin. Don't get discouraged. Keep working with your skin and be willing to adjust as needed.

CHAPTER 6

Common Myths

In the world of skincare, there are tons of common myths being spread around by enthusiasts, aficionados, and even some professionals! These myths can range from harmless to downright dangerous, so before we dive into skincare specifics and recommendations in the latter half of this book, let's address some common ones so you can develop an effective skincare regimen tailored to the specific needs of your melanated skin. Here are some common myths surrounding Black skincare:

Melanated skin doesn't need sunscreen: A common misconception is that darker skin tones are immune to sun damage. While melanin provides some natural protection, melanated skin can still experience sunburn, hyperpigmentation, and an increased risk of skin cancer without sunscreen.

Melanated skin doesn't age: Though melanin skin tends to show wrinkles later due to its thicker dermis and higher levels of collagen; it is still prone to aging concerns like hyperpigmentation, sagging, and uneven texture over time.

Oily skin doesn't need moisturizer: Many believe that because Black melanin skin can be oily, it doesn't require moisturizing. However, hydration is essential for all skin types, and skipping moisturizer can actually lead to more oil production as the skin tries to compensate for dryness.

Natural products are always better for Melanated skin: While natural ingredients can be beneficial, they can also cause irritation or allergic reactions. Melanin skin, like any skin type, requires careful selection of ingredients based on individual sensitivities.

Melanated skin doesn't scar: This is false, as Melanin skin is more prone to certain types of scarring like keloids and hyperpigmentation, especially after acne or injuries. It's important to treat wounds and breakouts early to minimize scarring.

Acne in melanin skin is always caused by oily skin: Acne can be caused by various factors such as hormones, bacteria, and inflammation, not just oily skin. Dry skin types can also experience breakouts due to irritation or product buildup.

Exfoliating frequently is necessary for smooth skin: Over-exfoliating can damage Black skin and worsen issues like hyperpigmentation. It's essential to balance exfoliation with gentle care to avoid irritation.

With these myths in mind, you can move forward on your skincare journey with the confidence to know you're doing what's best for your melanated skin.

CHAPTER 7

Building a Solid Foundation: The Essentials of a Good Skincare Regimen

A good skincare regimen doesn't have to be complicated or expensive, but it does need to be consistent and well-suited to your skin's unique needs. For folks with melanin-rich skin, this foundation is especially important because our skin has distinct characteristics that require specific care. From achieving balance to minimizing hyperpigmentation, there are foundational steps that will help you build an effective, everyday routine. In this chapter, I have provided the key essentials to incorporate into your regimen for healthier, glowing skin. It's recommended that you follow each of these steps in the order they are listed for the best results, but I understand if you need to skip a step to save money or time. Do the best you can, and remember that skincare is a lifelong journey.

Step 1: Cleanse

Cleansing is the cornerstone of any skincare regimen. A good cleanser will remove dirt, oil, makeup, and other impurities that accumulate on your skin throughout the day. Generally, regardless of your skin type, it is best to opt for a gentle, sulfate-free cleanser that won't strip your skin of its natural oils. Look for ingredients like glycerin or hyaluronic acid, which help retain moisture, and avoid products with harsh fragrances or alcohol that can cause irritation. It's important to note that using a face towel for cleansing is generally not recommended, as it can spread bacteria and irritate sensitive skin. Most experts advise using your hands or a designated soft washcloth for a gentler and more hygienic approach to cleansing.

Cleansing morning and night keeps your skin fresh and prepares it to absorb the next products in your routine. For nighttime cleansing, consider using a double-cleansing method if you wear makeup or sunscreen. This involves first using an oil-based cleanser to dissolve makeup, followed by a water-based cleanser to remove impurities. This two-step process ensures a deep clean without disrupting your skin's natural barrier. I personally use a Korean cleansing balm called "Clean It Zero," before using a gentle cleanser, nightly. This product pulls out all oil and grime while dissolving stubborn makeup and sunscreen.

Step 2: Tone

Toning helps balance your skin's pH after cleansing and removes any lingering impurities. While toners have evolved over the years, their role in hydration and preparing the skin for subsequent products remains essential. For melanated skin, which can be more prone to hyperpigmentation, a toner with gentle exfoliating acids like glycolic or lactic acid can help brighten the skin and fade dark spots over time. However, if your skin is sensitive, look for hydrating toners with ingredients like rose water, chamomile, or aloe vera.

Apply toner using a cotton pad or your fingertips, gently pressing it into the skin rather than rubbing. This step not only refreshes your skin but also enhances the absorption of serums and moisturizers. As a general note, it is not necessary to wait for your toner to dry completely before applying a serum, but if your toner contains active ingredients like glycolic or salicylic acid, you may want to wait to let them fully absorb to prevent layering irritation, especially if your serum contains other active ingredients.

Step 3: Treat (Serum)

Serums are concentrated formulas that target specific skin concerns, from acne and hyperpigmentation to fine lines and dryness. For those with hyperpigmentation, a vitamin C serum can be a great addition, as it is known for its brightening properties and ability to even skin tone. If you're dealing with acne or frequent breakouts, a serum with salicylic acid or niacin-amide can help control oil production, unclog pores, and reduce inflammation. Hyaluronic acid is an excellent all-rounder for hydration, suitable for all skin types, as it keeps skin plump and moisturized without feeling heavy.

Skin serums are typically applied twice a day—in the morning and in the evening—depending on the type of serum and its active ingredients. In the morning, it's best to use antioxidant serums like vitamin C and hydrating serums like hyaluronic acid. In the evening, it's best to use exfoliating serums like AHAs and BHAs, anti-aging serums like retinol, and repairing serums like niacin-amide.

When using serums, be sure to apply them before heavier products like moisturizers to maximize absorption. Like any other product, always test new serums to check for any potential irritation, and use sunscreen during the day, especially if you're applying serums with actives like vitamin C or retinol.

Step 4: Moisturize

No matter your skin type, moisturizer is essential. It seals in the benefits of your previous products, provides a protective barrier, and keeps your skin hydrated. For oily or acne-prone skin, opt for a lightweight, oil-free moisturizer that won't clog pores. If you have dry or combination skin, look for a thicker cream with ingredients like shea butter, ceramides, or squalane for extra hydration.

Don't skip moisturizer thinking it will make oily skin worse. Hydrating your skin well can actually help balance oil production. Melanated skin tends to lose moisture quickly, so this step is critical to maintaining that natural glow and preventing premature signs of aging.

To ensure your moisturizer performs at its best, always apply it to clean skin. For better absorption, it's preferable that you apply moisturizer when your skin is slightly damp. You can lightly mist your face with water after your other steps to accomplish this. Additionally, it's important that you start with a pea-sized amount—just enough to cover your face and neck without overloading—as using too much can clog your pores. When applying moisturizer, use gentle, upward strokes to spread the product over your face and neck without contributing to premature sagging and aging.

Moisturizers should generally be applied twice daily—once in the morning with a lightweight moisturizer after cleansing and before sunscreen, and once in the evening with a richer, hydrating formula to lock in moisture overnight. If you're experiencing especially dry or dehydrated skin throughout the day, you can apply more as needed.

Step 5: Sunscreen
Sunscreen is arguably the most important step in any skincare routine, yet it's often the most overlooked, especially for melanated skin. The truth is our melanin provides some natural protection against UV rays, but it's not enough to prevent sun damage, hyperpigmentation, or the risk of skin cancer. Use a broad-spectrum sunscreen with at least SPF 30 every day, even on cloudy days or when indoors, as UV rays can penetrate clouds and windows.

There are now many sunscreens formulated for deeper skin tones that won't leave a white cast. Look for mineral sunscreens with ingredients like zinc oxide or titanium dioxide, or chemical sunscreens that absorb well into the skin. Regular sunscreen use not only protects your skin from sun damage but also helps prevent dark spots from getting darker, ensuring a more even, radiant complexion.

When applying sunscreen, be sure to apply it generously every morning, even on cloudy days, using about a nickel-sized amount for your face and a shot-glass-sized amount for your entire body, at least fifteen to thirty minutes before going outside to allow it to absorb. Spread it evenly over all exposed areas, including your face, ears, neck, and the back of your hands, and reapply it every two hours, or more often if you're sweating or swimming.

Building Consistency in Your Routine

Skincare is a journey, and results don't happen overnight. Stick to a routine that feels manageable and sustainable, even if it's as simple as cleanse, moisturize, and protect with sunscreen. Over time, you'll see that the consistency of these steps is more effective than trying every new product on the market.

Remember, your skin may have different needs at different times of the year, or even at different times of the month if your breakouts are hormonal. Adjust your routine as needed, but keep these essentials at its core. The goal is to create a regimen that supports your skin's natural health, boosts confidence, and enhances your unique beauty.

CHAPTER 8

Revealing Radiance – A Guide to Retinol for Melanated Skin

In the world of skincare, retinoids are often considered a gold standard for treating a multitude of concerns. From acne to anti-aging, these vitamin A derivatives can transform the skin if used correctly. However, for those with melanin-rich skin, retinol can be a bit tricky to navigate. When used improperly, it can cause irritation, which may lead to hyperpigmentation. Retinoid and Retin-A (tretinoin) are two of the most well-known retinoids, but what exactly sets them apart? In this chapter, we'll break down the differences between the two and help you decide which one might be best for your skincare journey.

What Is Retinol?
Retinol has a reputation for being one of the most transformative skincare ingredients. Known for its ability to improve skin texture, minimize fine lines, and tackle stubborn hyperpigmentation, it can be a valuable addition to any skincare routine. Retinol is a form of

vitamin A that penetrates the outer layer of skin and reaches the middle layer, where it triggers cell turnover and stimulates collagen production, helping skin shed dead cells more rapidly. By boosting collagen production and skin renewal, retinol helps unclog pores and reduce the appearance of fine lines, improve skin texture, and even out pigmentation.

With regular use, it can leave your skin looking brighter, smoother, and more youthful; however, because melanated skin is more prone to inflammation, improper use of retinol can lead to irritation, which may cause hyperpigmentation. For this reason, it's essential to approach retinol carefully, starting with a lower concentration and gradually increasing usage over time. Whether you choose Retinol or Retin-A, both will help rejuvenate your skin, but their potency and how they work differ significantly.

Retin-A: The Gentle Giant

Retin-A is an over-the-counter (OTC) retinoid, meaning you can buy it without a prescription. It's considered the "gentler" cousin of Retin-A because it has to go through a conversion process before becoming active in your skin. When you apply retinol, your skin has to convert it into retinoic acid, which is the form that makes changes at the cellular level.

Pros:

- Gentler on the Skin: Because Retin-A is weaker than Retinoid (tretinoin), it's less likely to cause the irritation, redness, and peeling often associated with stronger retinoids.
- Widely Available: You can find retinol in many forms, from serums to creams, at different price points.
- Perfect for Beginners: If you're new to retinoids, retinol can be a great entry point to ease your skin into the powerful effects of vitamin A derivatives.

Cons:

- Takes Time to See Results: Since retinol must be converted into retinoic acid, the process can take time—often several months before you notice significant changes.
- Less Potent: While this gentleness can be a benefit, it also means that retinol might not be as effective for more stubborn skin issues, like severe acne or deep wrinkles.

Retin-A (Tretinoin): The Prescription Powerhouse

Retin-A, also known by its generic name, tretinoin, is a prescription-strength retinoid. Unlike retinol, it doesn't require any conversion. It's already in its active form as retinoic acid, which means it starts working on your skin as soon as you apply it. Because it's more potent, it's often recommended for more severe cases of acne, signs of aging, or hyperpigmentation.

Pros:

- Faster Results: Since Retin-A is more potent, it works faster than retinol. You might see changes in your skin in as little as six to eight weeks.
- More Effective: For those with serious acne or noticeable signs of aging, Retin-A can produce more dramatic results compared to retinol.
- Clinically Proven: Retin-A has been extensively studied and has a long history of being used successfully to treat a variety of skin concerns, especially acne.

Cons:

- Irritation is Common: Because of its strength, Retin-A can be quite irritating to the skin. Redness, peeling, and dryness are common side effects, especially in the early stages of use.
- Prescription Required: Unlike retinol, you'll need to visit a dermatologist to get a prescription for Retin-A.
- Not for the Faint of Heart: Retin-A requires a commitment to sun protection and a consistent skincare routine, as it can make your skin more sensitive to the sun.

Which One Should You Choose?

The choice between Retinol and Retin-A largely depends on your skin type, concerns, and how much time you have to dedicate to skincare.

Choose Retinol if:
- You have sensitive or dry skin.
- You're new to using retinoids and want to start with something gentler.
- You're looking for gradual, long-term improvements in texture, tone, and fine lines.

Choose Retin-A if:
- You have moderate to severe acne or signs of aging.
- You've used retinol before and are ready to move on to something stronger.
- You want quicker, more noticeable results and are okay with the possibility of some irritation.

Benefits of Retinol for Melanated Skin

Retinol can be highly beneficial for melanin-rich skin when used correctly. Here's how it can help:
- Evens Skin Tone: By promoting faster cell turnover, retinol can help fade hyperpigmentation, acne scars, and dark spots over time.
- Reduces Fine Lines and Wrinkles: Retinol boosts collagen production, which can help maintain skin elasticity and reduce the appearance of fine lines.
- Minimizes Acne and Breakouts: Retinol can help keep pores clear by exfoliating dead skin cells, reducing breakouts and acne scarring.

- Improves Skin Texture: Regular use of retinol can create a smoother, more refined texture, giving skin a healthy glow.
- Prevents Future Signs of Aging: By increasing cell turnover and collagen, retinol can help prevent premature aging and keep skin looking youthful.

With consistent, gradual use, retinol can be transformative for melanated skin. While results may take a few months to become visible, the long-term benefits are worth the patience and commitment.

Retinol can be intimidating, especially if you're worried about hyperpigmentation or irritation. But when used carefully, it can be a powerful ally in your skincare journey. Remember to be patient with your skin, and don't rush the process. The goal is to create a routine that enhances your natural beauty and celebrates the unique resilience of melanin-rich skin.

Choosing the Right Retinol for Melanin Skin

Finding the right retinol is essential for those with darker skin tones. Here are some key factors to look for:

- Low Concentrations: Start with a low-strength retinol (0.25% to 0.5%) to minimize the risk of irritation. Higher concentrations may cause peeling and sensitivity, which can lead to hyperpigmentation.

- Retinol Alternatives: Consider gentler forms of retinoids like retinaldehyde or retinyl palmitate, which offer similar benefits with less risk of irritation.
- Encapsulated Retinol: Encapsulated retinol is gradually released into the skin, reducing irritation while still delivering benefits. This makes it a great option for sensitive or melanin-rich skin.
- Added Soothing Ingredients: Look for retinol products with calming ingredients like niacinamide, hyaluronic acid, and ceramides. These ingredients help hydrate and soothe the skin, balancing retinol's potential drying effects.

Recommended Retinol Products for Melanin Skin

Here are some retinol products that work well for darker skin tones due to their gentle formulations and added hydrating ingredients:

- CeraVe Resurfacing Retinol Serum: This serum contains encapsulated retinol along with niacinamide and ceramides, making it gentle and safe for those with melanin-rich skin. It's great for evening out skin tone and fading dark spots.
- Murad Retinol Youth Renewal Serum: This serum uses a time-released retinol combined with hydrating and soothing ingredients like hyaluronic acid, reducing the chance of irritation. It's effective for tackling fine lines and promoting an even tone.
- Paula's Choice 0.3% Retinol + 2% Bakuchiol Treatment: This product combines a low concentration of retinol with

bakuchiol, a plant-based retinol alternative that further reduces irritation. It's a great choice for those new to retinol who want gradual benefits without risking sensitivity.
- The Ordinary Granactive Retinoid 2% Emulsion: This formula offers a gentle approach to retinol, using granactive retinoid instead of traditional retinol. It's effective for hyperpigmentation and uneven texture while being less likely to cause irritation.
- Shani Darden Retinol Reform: Created by celebrity esthetician Shani Darden, this retinol is known for its gentle yet effective formulation. It combines retinol with lactic acid, helping to smooth and brighten skin without over-drying.

How to Introduce Retinol Safely

Whether you choose retinol or Retin-A, there are some basic guidelines you should follow to get the most out of your product without damaging your skin:
- Start Slow: For both retinol and Retin-A, it's best to begin with a lower concentration of retinol and sparing use of just once or twice a week. As your skin builds tolerance, you can increase the frequency.
- Apply on Dry Skin: Wait for fifteen to twenty minutes after cleansing before applying retinol. Applying it to damp skin can increase absorption and potential irritation.

- Follow with a Moisturizer: Use a fragrance-free moisturizer after applying retinol to keep the skin hydrated and prevent dryness.
- Don't Mix with Exfoliants: Avoid using other exfoliating products (like AHAs, BHAs, or physical scrubs) on the same day as retinol to prevent over-exfoliating and irritating your skin.
- Sun Protection is a Must: This is non-negotiable. Retinoids make your skin more sensitive to the sun, so wearing a broad-spectrum SPF 30 or higher daily is crucial to avoid sunburns and further damage.
- Be Patient: Even with Retin-A, you won't see overnight results. Stick with your routine for at least eight to twelve weeks to see noticeable changes.
- Consult a Dermatologist: If you're unsure which retinoid is right for you, or if you experience significant irritation, it's always a good idea to seek professional advice.

Managing Retinol Side Effects

Even with a cautious approach, it's normal to experience some initial dryness, redness, or peeling when starting retinol. Here's how to manage these side effects:

- Hydrate Regularly: Apply a moisturizer with hydrating ingredients like hyaluronic acid, glycerin, or ceramides after retinol to lock in moisture.

- Consider "Buffering": If retinol feels too intense, you can try "buffering" it by mixing it with a moisturizer before applying it to your skin. This dilutes the strength slightly and makes it gentler.
- Use Barrier-Strengthening Products: Ingredients like niacinamide and squalane help maintain the skin's natural barrier and reduce sensitivity.
- Adjust Your Routine as Needed: If you notice peeling or irritation, reduce your usage frequency. It's okay to take a break from retinol for a week or so if your skin needs recovery time.

Both retinol and Retin-A are incredibly powerful tools for improving the health and appearance of your skin, but they serve different purposes. Retinol is ideal for those who want a gentler approach with gradual results, while Retin-A is perfect for those looking for faster and more dramatic changes. By understanding the strengths and limitations of each, you can make an informed choice and achieve your best skin yet.

In the end, the best skincare routine is one that suits your skin's needs and fits your lifestyle. Whether you go with retinol or Retin-A, consistency and care are key. Remember, skincare is a journey, not a race—so take your time and find what works best for you. Retinol is just one tool, but it's a potent one that, when used wisely, can bring out the very best in your skin. Embrace the process, stay consistent, and watch your skin reveal its natural radiance.

CHAPTER 9

The Magic of Moisturizing for Melanin-Rich Skin

Moisturizing is an essential step for all skin types, but it carries unique significance for melanin-rich skin. Due to its natural ability to retain more moisture, melanin-rich skin can sometimes mask dehydration issues until they become more prominent. However, it also has a heightened sensitivity to certain ingredients and environmental factors, making a balanced, hydrating skincare routine crucial. There are a few reasons why moisturizing matters, particularly for melanin-rich skin. Let's take a look at a few.

First, moisturizing prevents hyperpigmentation. As we've learned, melanin-rich skin is more prone to hyperpigmentation and discoloration when irritated, and a well-moisturized skin barrier is less susceptible to inflammation and irritation, which can help reduce the likelihood of dark spots forming after a breakout or scratch. Moisturizing also helps maintain the skin barrier, which acts as a shield against pollutants and harmful UV rays. When melanin-rich skin is dehydrated, it can lead to a weakened barrier that is less effective at protecting against damage, dryness, and other irritants.

Many people with melanin-rich skin produce more natural oils, which can lead to a misconception that skipping moisturizer is beneficial. However, hydrating with the right moisturizer balances natural oil production, leading to smoother and healthier skin without clogging pores. And finally, moisturizing combats aging. Although melanin-rich skin is more resistant to visible signs of aging, that doesn't make it immune. The effects of aging, such as loss of elasticity and dullness, can be minimized by a consistent moisturizing routine.

Key Ingredients to Look for in a Moisturizer

When choosing a moisturizer for melanin-rich skin, certain ingredients can elevate the skin's hydration while ensuring it remains balanced and protected.

- Hyaluronic Acid: Holds up to 1,000 times its weight in water, making it ideal for intense hydration.
- Niacinamide (Vitamin B3): Reduces redness and inflammation, helping with skin tone and texture. Niacinamide can also reduce the appearance of dark spots.
- Shea Butter: Naturally rich in vitamins and fatty acids, shea butter is a powerhouse for moisturizing without clogging pores, which is ideal for melanin- rich skin.
- Ceramides: Essential for skin barrier health, ceramides lock in moisture and provide a layer of protection against environmental pollutants.

- Glycerin: This humectant attracts water to the skin's surface, keeping it supple and hydrated.

Recommended Moisturizers for Melanin-Rich Skin

CeraVe Daily Moisturizing Lotion

Best For: All skin types, especially sensitive skin.

Why: This affordable and gentle moisturizer is packed with ceramides and hyaluronic acid. It provides long-lasting hydration without leaving a greasy feel and is fragrance-free, making it ideal for sensitive skin.

Fenty Skin Hydra Vizor Invisible Moisturizer + SPF 30

Best For: Daily wear with sun protection.

Why: Created by Rihanna, this moisturizer includes SPF protection, is light enough for daily wear, and works well under makeup. It is packed with niacinamide to brighten the skin and fight hyperpigmentation while keeping it hydrated.

La Roche-Posay Toleriane Double Repair Face Moisturizer

Best For: Sensitive and acne-prone skin.

Why: This moisturizer contains prebiotic thermal water, ceramides, and niacinamide. It helps to repair and protect the skin barrier, soothe irritation, and prevent the dryness that can lead to ashy tones on darker skin.

Shea Moisture African Black Soap Balancing Moisturizer

Best For: Oily or acne-prone skin.

Why: This moisturizer contains shea butter, which is excellent for hydration, along with tea tree oil to balance oil production. It's especially beneficial for those dealing with acne and discoloration, as it hydrates without clogging pores.

First Aid Beauty Ultra Repair Cream

Best For: Dry and eczema-prone skin.

Why: Known for its deeply hydrating properties, this cream is ideal for very dry skin. It's formulated with colloidal oatmeal, which calms irritation and works well on melanin-rich skin prone to dryness and sensitivity.

Youth to the People Superfood Air-Whip Moisture Cream

Best For: Combination skin.

Why: This cream is light but deeply hydrating, making it perfect for combination skin. It's packed with antioxidant-rich ingredients like kale and green tea, helping to fight free radicals while keeping the skin moisturized.

Moisturizing Tips for Melanin-Rich Skin

- Layer for Hydration: After cleansing, apply a hydrating serum with hyaluronic acid before your moisturizer. This helps lock in moisture and keeps skin hydrated for longer.

- Don't Skip Night Moisturizing: Nighttime is when the skin regenerates and repairs itself. Using a slightly thicker or more nourishing moisturizer at night can make a significant difference in skin texture and brightness.
- SPF is Essential: Melanin-rich skin is not immune to sun damage. Using a moisturizer with SPF or applying SPF on top of your moisturizer can prevent hyperpigmentation and protect against aging.

Keeping your melanin-rich skin hydrated is key to achieving an even tone, preventing dryness, and maintaining its natural glow

Chapter 10

SPF, SPF, SPF!

One of the simplest and most effective things you can do for your skin, regardless of complexion, is to apply sunscreen daily. Specifically, a broad-spectrum sunscreen with SPF 30 or higher is essential for protecting your skin from the harmful effects of the sun. For melanin-rich skin, there's a common misconception that we don't need sunscreen because our natural pigment, melanin, provides some degree of sun protection. While it's true that melanin offers a natural defense against UV damage, it's far from enough to keep your skin fully protected.

Melanin does provide a bit of a barrier—darker skin tones are less prone to immediate sunburn and show slower signs of visible aging than lighter skin tones. However, this doesn't mean we're immune to sun damage. Regardless of how much melanin you have, UV radiation from the sun penetrates the skin, causing harm at deeper levels, even if we don't see or feel it right away. This damage can lead to long-term issues like hyperpigmentation, premature aging, and in more severe cases, skin cancer. In fact, studies have shown that Black individuals are often diagnosed with skin cancer at more advanced stages, largely because of the misconception that we aren't at risk.

For melanin-rich skin, the most obvious challenge from sun exposure is hyperpigmentation. UV rays can also worsen existing skin conditions like acne scars, eczema, or melasma, leaving marks that take longer to fade. Even if you have clear skin, not wearing sunscreen can cause discoloration over time, making it harder to achieve that even, glowing complexion we all strive for.

Applying sunscreen daily helps prevent this damage and ensures your skin stays protected no matter your level of exposure to the sun. Sunscreen acts as a shield, blocking both UVA rays (which cause aging) and UVB rays (which cause burning). By integrating it into your skincare routine, you not only prevent immediate sunburn but also keep your skin barrier strong, reduce inflammation, and minimize the risk of uneven tone and dark spots.

It's important to choose the right type of sunscreen for melanin-rich skin. Traditional sunscreens have a reputation for leaving a white cast, which is especially noticeable on darker skin tones. Thankfully, modern formulations, including tinted and mineral-based sunscreens, are designed with melanated skin in mind. These new options blend seamlessly into the skin, without leaving behind that ashy residue, so you can stay protected without compromising your appearance.

If you're wearing makeup, don't skip your SPF. Many foundations now come with built-in SPF, but relying solely on makeup with SPF isn't enough. You'll still need a dedicated sunscreen under your foundation to ensure full protection. If you're outdoors for extended periods, it's also a good idea to reapply it every two hours.

Incorporating sunscreen into your daily routine is an easy but powerful step. Whether it's a sunny day or cloudy, UV rays are always present. By making sunscreen a non-negotiable part of your skincare regimen, you're taking proactive steps toward protecting your skin's health, preserving your complexion, and preventing long-term damage. After all, one of the greatest acts of self-love for your skin is protecting it every day.

Recommended Sunscreen Options for Melanin-Rich Skin

When it comes to choosing the right sunscreen for melanin-rich skin, it's essential to find formulas that offer broad-spectrum protection without leaving a white cast. Here are some great options specifically designed to blend seamlessly with darker skin tones while providing optimal protection.

Black Girl Sunscreen SPF 30

Why it's great: Specifically created for dark skin tones, Black Girl Sunscreen is a lightweight, moisturizing sunscreen that doesn't leave any white residue. It's infused with natural ingredients like avocado, jojoba, and carrot juice, which help hydrate the skin and even out skin tone.

Perfect for: Daily use under makeup or alone for a fresh, natural look

Supergoop! Unseen Sunscreen SPF 40

Why it's great: This invisible, weightless sunscreen is perfect for melanin-rich skin. It's oil-free and works well for all skin types, including oily and acne-prone skin. It also doubles as a makeup primer, making it versatile for everyday use.

Perfect for: A matte finish and those looking for a primer-sunscreen combo

Color Science Sunforgettable Total Protection Face Shield SPF 50 (Bronze or Glow)

Why it's great: This tinted mineral sunscreen provides broad-spectrum protection and is available in shades that blend perfectly into melanin-rich skin. The lightweight formula not only shields against UVA/UVB rays but also defends against environmental factors like pollution and blue light.

Perfect for: Those looking for a tinted sunscreen that offers additional environmental protection and leaves no white cast

La Roche-Posay Anthelios Melt-in Milk Sunscreen SPF 100

Why it's great: With high-level, broad-spectrum protection, this sunscreen is perfect for those who want maximum defense. The "melt-in milk" formula absorbs quickly without leaving an ashy or greasy residue.

Perfect for: Extended sun exposure, such as outdoor activities or beach days

EltaMD UV Clear Broad-Spectrum SPF 46

Why it's great: Dermatologist-recommended for sensitive, acne-prone, or oily skin, this sheer formula absorbs quickly without a white cast. It contains niacinamide to reduce inflammation and promote even skin tone.

Perfect for: Sensitive or acne-prone skin, or those dealing with hyperpigmentation

Fenty Skin Hydra Vizor Invisible Moisturizer Broad Spectrum SPF 30

Why it's great: Designed by Rihanna, this lightweight sunscreen doubles as a moisturizer, blends seamlessly into melanin-rich skin, and leaves no white residue.

Perfect for: Daily use as a moisturizer and sunscreen combo

CeraVe Hydrating Mineral Sunscreen SPF 30

Why it's great: This lightweight, mineral sunscreen is gentle on the skin and blends better than most mineral formulas. It's fragrance-free and non-comedogenic, making it a great option for sensitive skin.

Perfect for: Dry or sensitive skin types

Neutrogena Hydro Boost Water Gel Lotion SPF 30

Why it's great: With a light, hydrating formula, this sunscreen absorbs like a water gel, leaving no greasy or ashy residue. It's ideal for daily use on darker skin tones.

Perfect for: Combination or dry skin types needing hydration

Bolden SPF 30 Brightening Moisturizer

Why it's great: From a Black-owned brand, this sunscreen is formulated to help even skin tone while offering sun protection. It's a great option for those looking to prevent and treat dark spots.

Perfect for: Daily use, especially for those dealing with hyperpigmentation

Unsun Mineral Tinted Sunscreen SPF 30

Why it's great: Created specifically for people of color, Unsun offers a mineral-based, tinted sunscreen that blends well into medium to deep skin tones without leaving a white cast.

Perfect for: Those looking for light makeup coverage along with sun protection

Aveeno Positively Mineral Sensitive Skin Sunscreen SPF 50

Why it's great: This sunscreen is gentle, lightweight, and formulated for sensitive skin. It contains soothing oat, and though it's a mineral-based sunscreen, it blends well on darker skin tones.

Perfect for: Sensitive skin needing high SPF protection

By incorporating one of these sunscreens into your daily skincare routine, you'll be protecting your melanin-rich skin from sun damage, preventing hyperpigmentation, and keeping your complexion healthy and even-toned.

Chapter 11

Feed Your Skin: The Power of Nutrition and Health for a Balanced Life

When it comes to skin health, what you put on your plate can be just as important as what you put on your skin. Nourishing your body from the inside with a balanced diet and a healthy lifestyle provides the essential nutrients that promote a glowing, resilient complexion. In this chapter, we'll explore the connection between nutrition, skin health, and overall wellness, and how to create a balanced lifestyle that supports not only beautiful skin but also a vibrant, energized you.

The Skin-Nutrition Connection
Our skin reflects what's going on inside our bodies. Nutrient-rich foods provide the building blocks for skin cells, help balance hormones, and support the immune system. Poor nutrition, on the other hand, can contribute to inflammation, dehydration, and

premature aging. That's why a healthy, balanced diet is one of the best skincare products you can invest in.

Key nutrients play specific roles in maintaining skin health. For example, vitamin C supports collagen production, while antioxidants combat damage from free radicals, which contribute to aging. Omega-3 fatty acids keep skin supple and hydrated, while zinc helps reduce inflammation and promote healing. Together, these nutrients create a foundation for clear, resilient skin.

Building a Balanced Diet for Radiant Skin

A balanced diet is not about strict rules or deprivation, but rather about enjoying a variety of foods that give your body what it needs to thrive. Here are some dietary principles that support both skin and overall health:

- Eat the Rainbow: Fill your plate with a variety of colorful fruits and vegetables. Each color represents different nutrients that are vital for skin health. For example, oranges and peppers are rich in vitamin C, which supports collagen, while leafy greens provide vitamin E, a powerful antioxidant.
- Healthy Fats Are Your Friend: Healthy fats, like those found in avocados, nuts, seeds, and olive oil, help keep skin hydrated and supple. Omega-3 fatty acids, found in salmon, chia seeds, and flax seeds, are particularly beneficial for reducing inflammation and promoting a smooth, plump appearance.

- Protein Power: Protein is essential for cell repair and growth, which makes it critical for skin health. Lean meats, fish, beans, and legumes are excellent sources. Collagen-rich foods, like bone broth, can also support skin elasticity.
- Hydrate for Glow: Water is vital for healthy skin, as it keeps cells hydrated, helps flush out toxins, and prevents dryness. Aim to drink plenty of water throughout the day, and incorporate hydrating foods, like cucumbers, watermelon, and leafy greens, into your diet.
- Limit Sugary and Processed Foods: Sugar and processed foods can contribute to inflammation, breakouts, and premature aging. When you eat sugar, it triggers a process called glycation, which damages collagen and elastin in the skin. Opt for natural sweeteners, like honey or fruit, when you need a sweet treat.
- Prioritize Gut Health: A healthy gut promotes clear, balanced skin. Fermented foods like yogurt, kimchi, and sauerkraut support the growth of beneficial bacteria in your gut, which can reduce inflammation and improve your skin's appearance. Adding fiber-rich foods like whole grains, fruits, and vegetables also supports digestive health.

Foods That Specifically Benefit Skin

While all whole foods support your health, certain foods are particularly beneficial for your skin:

- Berries: Rich in antioxidants, especially vitamin C, berries protect skin from environmental damage and support collagen production.
- Leafy Greens: Spinach, kale, and collard greens are packed with vitamins A, C, and E, which support skin repair and protect against free radicals.
- Nuts and Seeds: Almonds, walnuts, and sunflower seeds are great sources of vitamin E, an antioxidant that helps prevent skin aging.
- Sweet Potatoes and Carrots: High in beta-carotene, which your body converts into vitamin A, these vegetables help promote a healthy skin tone and may reduce acne.
- Fatty Fish: Salmon, mackerel, and sardines are rich in omega-3 fatty acids, which reduce inflammation and keep skin hydrated and supple.

Balancing Your Lifestyle for Radiant Skin

Skin health goes beyond just what you eat. A balanced lifestyle supports your skin, energy, and well-being:

- Prioritize Sleep: Your skin repairs itself while you sleep. A lack of rest can lead to dullness, fine lines, and dark circles. Aim seven to eight hours of quality sleep each night, and establish a calming bedtime routine to promote rest.
- Manage Stress: Stress triggers the release of cortisol, a hormone that can lead to inflammation, breakouts, and an overall lackluster complexion. Practice stress-reducing

activities like meditation, deep breathing, or spending time in nature. Prioritizing self-care is a powerful way to support both your mind and skin.

- Exercise Regularly: Physical activity improves circulation, which delivers oxygen and nutrients to your skin cells, giving you a natural glow. Exercise also helps manage stress, supporting hormonal balance and overall well-being. Find activities you enjoy, whether it's dancing, hiking, or yoga.
- Avoid Smoking and Excessive Alcohol: Smoking and alcohol dehydrate the skin and accelerate aging. Smoking decreases blood flow to the skin, while alcohol depletes vitamin A and can cause puffiness. If you drink alcohol, do so in moderation and stay hydrated.
- Practice Sun Protection: UV rays are one of the leading causes of skin aging.
- Wear SPF 30 or higher daily, even on cloudy days. Sun protection prevents hyperpigmentation, fine lines, and other signs of aging, allowing your skin's natural beauty to shine through.

The Power of Consistency

Consistency is the key to achieving and maintaining radiant skin. Just as a single healthy meal won't transform your health, long-term, sustainable habits are necessary for meaningful changes. Approach your diet and lifestyle with a sense of balance and flexibility. It's okay to enjoy treats or take a day off from exercise. The goal is to create habits that are enjoyable and sustainable in the long run.

Embracing Self-Love Through Nutrition and Health

A balanced diet and lifestyle are about more than just appearances; they're a form of self-respect and self-love. Nourishing your body with wholesome foods, staying active, and managing stress are ways to care for yourself from the inside out. When you treat your body well, it shows in your skin and your overall radiance. Remember that taking care of your skin isn't just about products; it's about honoring yourself with nourishing choices and habits that let your natural beauty shine. Embrace the journey of learning what makes you feel your best, and let that inner glow radiate through your skin.

CHAPTER 12

The Sun, Vitamin D, and Melanin Skin

When it comes to skincare, one of the most misunderstood topics is the role of sunlight and vitamin D in our skin's health, especially for those of us with melanated skin. Although I've spent quite a bit of time in this book warning you against the harms of the sum, vitamin D is essential for our bodies, as it supports our immune system, bone health, and even mood regulation. But for skin of color, which naturally has more melanin, our relationship with the sun and vitamin D production is a bit more complex.

Understanding Melanin and Sun Exposure
Melanin is what gives skin its color, and the more melanin you have, the deeper your natural skin tone. Melanin is also your skin's natural protector against harmful UV rays, which can lead to premature aging, sunburn, and skin cancer. Think of melanin as a shield, working to absorb and disperse UV rays so that less damage reaches your skin cells. But while this built-in sun protection can be

beneficial, it also has an impact on how well our skin produces vitamin D.

Vitamin D is often called the "sunshine vitamin" because our bodies produce it when exposed to sunlight, specifically UVB rays. However, melanin can make it more challenging for these UVB rays to penetrate the skin, meaning that those of us with more melanin require more sun exposure to produce adequate levels of vitamin D. For those with lighter skin, as little as ten to fifteen minutes of sun exposure a few times a week might be enough, but people with darker skin tones often need much more time outdoors—sometimes up to three times as much.

The Importance of Vitamin D for Melanin Skin

Vitamin D does a lot more than just support bone health; it also plays a vital role in maintaining skin health, too. This nutrient can help regulate cell turnover, which is essential for preventing issues like hyperpigmentation and inflammation, both of which can be more common concerns in melanated skin. Vitamin D also has anti-inflammatory properties that can soothe skin conditions such as eczema and acne. If you're dealing with breakouts or irritation, making sure you are taking in enough vitamin D might help calm things down, controlling inflammation and reducing redness and flare-ups.

Low levels of vitamin D, however, are common in people of color. When the body doesn't receive enough, like during the cold dark months of winter, it can sometimes lead to issues like dry skin, eczema, and other inflammatory skin conditions. Since melanated skin already faces unique challenges in maintaining an even skin tone and texture, a vitamin D deficiency can add to those issues, making it essential for us to find ways to ensure adequate intake.

Safely Soaking Up the Sun

So, how can you get enough vitamin D without risking sun damage? Here are a few tips to help you balance sun exposure and skin protection:

- Smart Sun Time: Aim for shorter bursts of sun exposure during off-peak hours (before 10 a.m. or after 4 p.m.), especially if you're prone to dark spots or hyperpigmentation. A short walk in the sun for fifteen to twenty minutes a few times a week can help boost vitamin D levels without excessive UV exposure.
- Don't Skip Sunscreen: Even though melanin provides some natural protection, it's still essential to wear sunscreen daily. Opt for a broad-spectrum sunscreen with at least SPF 30. This will help prevent UV damage, premature aging, and hyperpigmentation. Look for mineral sunscreens with zinc oxide or titanium dioxide, as they're often less irritating to melanated skin.
- Dietary Sources and Supplements: If you don't get much sun exposure or want to avoid it, you can get vitamin D from food sources like fatty fish (salmon, tuna, mackerel), fortified milk, and orange juice. Supplements are also an effective

option but be sure to consult with a healthcare provider to determine the right dosage for your skin and body.
- Regular Vitamin D Check-Ups: Consider getting your vitamin D levels tested, especially if you don't get much sun exposure. Many people with melanated skin don't realize they're deficient, and knowing your levels can guide you in making better decisions for your skin and health.

Embracing a Holistic Approach to Sun and Skin Health

Taking care of melanated skin is about embracing a holistic approach. While vitamin D is essential, it's only one part of the puzzle. Balancing sun exposure with sunscreen, eating nutrient-rich foods, and understanding your skin's unique needs all contribute to a healthier complexion. Protecting your skin doesn't mean avoiding the sun altogether but rather finding a balance that respects your skin's natural beauty and needs.

So, the next time you step outside, think of your relationship with the sun as an act of self-care and self-respect. Your skin deserves to glow from the inside out, nourished by both nature and science. By taking these steps, you can enjoy the benefits of vitamin D without compromising the health or beauty of your skin.

CHAPTER 13

Embracing Youthfulness: A Melanated Guide to Anti-Aging

Aging is a natural, beautiful part of life, and while our skin naturally changes over time, there's a lot we can do to keep it healthy, glowing, and resilient. Anti-aging isn't about stopping time; it's about nourishing our skin in ways that protect it, encourage cell renewal, and help us feel confident at every stage of life. In this chapter, we'll explore practices, ingredients, and routines that support youthful, radiant skin.

The Basics of Anti-Aging for Melanated Skin
Melanated skin has a unique set of needs and characteristics due to its higher melanin content. Melanin provides a natural defense against the sun's UV rays, which is one of the main causes of premature aging. However, this doesn't mean Black skin is immune to the effects of aging; rather, it ages in ways that are unique, like developing pigmentation changes, fine lines around the eyes, and a gradual loss of elasticity.

The key to anti-aging for Black skin involves a proactive, daily approach that protects and strengthens the skin's barrier. This includes consistent hydration, protection from environmental stressors, and adopting a lifestyle that reduces aging risk factors.

A simple, effective anti-aging routine focuses on cleansing, moisturizing, protecting, and targeting specific concerns. Here's a daily routine designed for youthful-looking skin:

- Gentle Cleansing: Start with a sulfate-free, hydrating cleanser. As skin ages, it can lose moisture more easily, so look for ingredients like ceramides, glycerin, and gentle botanical extracts that won't strip your skin of its natural oils.

- Exfoliate Regularly: Regular exfoliation removes dead skin cells that can make skin look dull and enhances cell turnover. For anti-aging, opt for gentle exfoliants like lactic acid or mandelic acid, rather than physical exfoliants like facial scrubs or sponges. These chemical exfoliators are less likely to irritate darker skin tones and can help brighten and smooth your skin.

- Hydrating Serums: Use serums that deliver antioxidants like vitamin C, vitamin E, and ferulic acid to protect against environmental stress. Hyaluronic acid is also ideal for boosting hydration, which helps keep the skin plump and reduces the appearance of fine lines. You can also opt for ingredients like niacinamide, licorice root extract, and alpha-arbutin to help fade dark spots. These can be used alongside your retinoid at night or a vitamin C serum in the morning to even skin tone and create a more radiant complexion.

- Moisturizing: A thicker moisturizer locks in hydration and supports the skin barrier. Look for options containing peptides, which support collagen production, and squalane, which mimics the skin's natural oils.
- Sun Protection: This is non-negotiable! Use a broad-spectrum SPF 30 or higher every day. For melanated skin, a mineral sunscreen with tinted formulas can prevent the white cast while protecting against UV rays.
- Nighttime Nourishment: In the evening, consider a retinoid or retinol product. Retinoids are known for their powerful anti-aging effects, helping to increase cell turnover, reduce hyperpigmentation, and promote collagen production. Always use retinoids with caution, starting with a low dose, and alternate nights to avoid irritation.

Lifestyle Tips for Anti-Aging

In addition to skincare, lifestyle changes can also help you maintain youthful skin:

- Eat for Skin Health: A diet rich in antioxidants, omega-3 fatty acids, and vitamins supports your skin from the inside out. Berries, leafy greens, fish, nuts, and whole grains are packed with nutrients that fight free radicals and promote skin elasticity.

- Stay Hydrated: Hydrated skin is healthy skin. Drinking plenty of water throughout the day helps flush out toxins and keeps skin cells plump.
- Reduce Stress: Stress can accelerate aging due to the release of cortisol, a hormone that can break down collagen. Regular exercise, meditation, and enough sleep are all powerful tools for managing stress and keeping skin vibrant.
- Sleep Well: Sleep is a time when the body repairs itself, including skin cells. Aim for seven to eight hours of rest every night to allow your skin to rejuvenate, reducing the risk of fine lines and dullness.

Anti-aging is less about changing how we look and more about caring for our skin in ways that let us feel our best. Our skin tells our story, and each line, mark, and feature is a part of who we are. The goal isn't perfection, but instead, embracing the journey and caring for our skin so it reflects our health, confidence, and vitality.

Conclusion

As we close this journey together, let's celebrate the progress you've made in understanding and caring for your skin. From learning about the unique needs of melanin-rich skin to discovering the best routines and products to address acne, hyperpigmentation, and overall skin health, you now have the tools to take control of your skincare journey.

But remember, this is just the beginning. Skin care is a lifelong commitment to self-love, patience, and growth. With consistency and care, you can continue to embrace your natural beauty and glow unapologetically.

This book is just one chapter in a larger story. I have so much more to share—about wellness, beauty, and the connection between self-care and confidence. Stay tuned, because there's more to come, and I can't wait to continue this journey with you.

Until then, keep loving yourself and your skin.

With love and gratitude,
Morgan

Acknowledgements

I extend my heartfelt gratitude to my wonderful cousin, author S.N.M Jones, whose intelligence and kindness have been a constant source of encouragement. I am deeply grateful to Dr. James Berman, MD, for his invaluable mentorship, expertise on skin conditions and treatments, and unwavering support. Lastly, to my parents, thank you for being my steadfast foundation and source of strength throughout this journey.

Made in the USA
Columbia, SC
04 April 2025